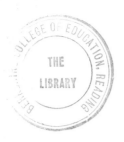

HUMAN PHYSIOLOGY

HUMAN PHYSIOLOGY
A PROGRAMMED TEXT

CERTIFIED MEDICAL REPRESENTATIVES INSTITUTE, INC.
Roanoke, Virginia

PREPARED BY

Psychological Consultants, Inc.
Richmond, Virginia

CONSULTANT

Robert E. Thurber, Ph.D
Associate Professor of Physiology
Jefferson Medical College
Philadelphia, Pennsylvania

JOHN WILEY & SONS, INC.   New York · London · Sydney · Toronto

PREFACE

Physiology is the study of the functions of living systems. A system might be a single cell, a particular organ, a group of organs, or an entire individual. In his study of how things work in a living organism, the physiologist uses the principles of mathematics, chemistry, and physics. Although anatomy emphasizes the structure of a living system and physiology emphasizes the functions and interrelations of these structures, both structure and function—anatomy and physiology—are inseparable if one is to understand the living system.

This physiology program is concerned with normal physiology; that is, it deals with the healthy individual. Excursions outside the normal limits of the physiological variables constitute disease, and if the control mechanisms of the body cannot return the system to its normal state, medical intervention is indicated. Treatment often consists of a specific drug therapy, the purpose being to return the body to a normal range of physiological activity.

For learning convenience we have divided this physiology program in accordance with the general systems of the body. It should be remembered that the systems do not function independently in the body; they form a well-integrated unit.

You will probably find that you will learn most effectively if you use the following procedures:

1. Read each item (or frame) carefully and completely.

2. Use the answer shield, or a similar card, to cover the responses (which appear just opposite the next frame) until you check your written response.

3. Always *write your responses,* which will help you remember more effectively and will also aid in the spelling of many technical terms. Then compare your response to the text response. Use your best judgment to decide whether your response is sufficiently similar to the text response to consider it a correct one.

4. If you believe that your response is incorrect or inadequate, place an X by the frame number, and then write the correct response. This should be an aid to you in reviewing the material later.

5. Go on to the next frame when you have made a correct response or after you have corrected a wrong response.

6. In the program there will be some information frames where responses are not required. In such instances, read the frame carefully and then go on to the next frame.

The time required to master the material will depend on your previous knowledge and background. The physiology program was pretested on a group of individuals who had varied backgrounds, and completion times averaged approximately twelve hours. There are review sections at the conclusion of the program which will give you an idea of the level of knowledge you are expected to attain. Review Number One covers Sections I and II of the program; Review Number Two covers Sections III and IV; Review Number Three covers Sections V, VI, and VII; and Review Number Four covers Section VIII. The correct answers for the questions are at the end of the review sections. It will be best to answer the review questions after you have completed the appropriate sections for each review. If you miss an item, be sure to re-study the related material.

Listed below are the major behavioral objectives for the physiology program. These can serve as a checklist to guide your study and as a measure of your accomplishment. If you study the program as indicated, you should be able to:

Section I

1. Define cell physiology.
2. List three types of extracellular fluids.
3. Differentiate between the normal and abnormal relations of a cell with its environment.
4. Describe and explain Fick's law.
5. Describe the action of the sodium pump.
6. Distinguish between isosmotic and isotonic solutions.
7. List the factors affecting the movement of a substance across the cell membrane.
8. Define diffusion, osmosis, osmotic pressure and isotonic solutions.

Section II

1. State Ohm's law.
2. Describe membrane potential.
3. List and define the refractory periods of the recovery stage of a nerve fiber.
4. Classify the three types of nerve fibers.
5. Describe the process of muscle cell contraction.
6. Describe conditions that block nerve-muscle transmission.

7. State the relationship of ATP to muscular contraction.
8. State the cause of maximum muscle contraction.
9. Name the parts of a motor unit.
10. Distinguish between isometric and isotonic contractions.
11. State the all-or-none law.
12. Define nerve impulse, rheobase, myelin sheath, axon, fibril, sarcomere, synapse, EPSP, and myasthenia gravis.

Section III

1. Differentiate between afferent and efferent nerves.
2. Sketch the path of a sensory impulse from the point of stimulation to the cortex.
3. Sketch the path of a motor impulse from the cortex to a muscle fiber.
4. Diagram a spinal reflex pathway.
5. Describe the mechanism of a stretch reflex.
6. Describe the mechanism of maintaining body balance.
7. Diagram the lens system of the eye.
8. List and describe refractive errors in vision.
9. Describe the process of visual accommodation.
10. Explain the mechanism of transfer of sound waves to a hearing experience.
11. Differentiate between the sympathetic and parasympathetic systems.
12. List the major portions of the brain.
13. Given a diagram of the brain, locate the reticular formation, thalamus, hypothalamus, cerebellum, the sensory area of the cerebrum, and the motor area of the cerebrum.
14. State the functions of each of the areas listed in item 13.
15. List the four lobes of the cerebrum.
16. Define sensory localization, receptor, reticular formation, muscle spindle, presbyopia, and ganglia.

Section IV

1. Describe the major constituents of blood.
2. Describe the formation of red blood cells.
3. Describe the mechanism of jaundice.
4. State the nature of blood plasma.
5. Describe the mechanism of blood clotting.
6. List techniques for the prevention of blood clotting.
7. Explain the ABO system of blood typing.
8. Describe the mechanism of blood flow.

9. Explain the mechanism of heart activity.
10. Differentiate between systole and diastole.
11. Describe the procedure for measuring blood pressure.
12. List ECG waves.
13. Explain the relationship between sympathetic and parasympathetic actions and the heart.
14. Describe the function of the lymphatic capillaries.
15. Define hemoglobin, carbonic anhydrase, cyanosis, erythrocyte, hypochromic anemia, aplastic anemia, pulmonary embolism, phagocytes, blood pressure, ECG (EKG), stenosis, fibrillation, and pressoreceptor reflex.

Section V

1. State the gas law.
2. Explain the diffusion of oxygen and carbon dioxide in the lungs.
3. List the forms by which carbon dioxide is transported in the blood.
4. Describe the mechanism of inspiration.
5. Diagram the factors affecting breathing.
6. Describe the relationship of the lungs to the regulation of acidity in the blood.
7. Describe the transfer of oxygen and carbon dioxide across the capillary walls.
8. Define carbamino compound, residual volume, and tidal volume.

Section VI

1. Describe the process of urine formation.
2. State the formula for the clearance of a substance in the plasma.
3. Describe the mechanism of bicarbonate conversion.
4. Describe the renal handling of ammonia.
5. Describe the renal regulation of blood pH.
6. Define glomerulus, nephron, glomerular filtration rate, plasma clearance, tubular maximum and diuresis.

Section VII

1. List the functions of saliva.
2. Describe the process of the digestion of fat.
3. Describe the mechanism of digestion and the movement of undigested food.
4. Define pepsin, gastrin, enterogastrone, secretin, pancreozymin.

Section VIII

1. Differentiate between endocrine and exocrine glands.
2. State the three classes of adrenal cortex hormones and the functions of each.
3. State the two hormones associated with the Islet cells of the pancreas and the functions of each.
4. State the two types of sex hormones produced by the ovaries and the functions of each.
5. Describe the mechanism of the menstrual cycle.
6. Describe the relationship of hormones to milk production in the mammary gland.
7. Define target gland.
8. Define goiter.
9. State the relationship of the endocrine glands of the body to the following hormones and the physiological function of each of the hormones: growth hormone, thyrotrophic hormone, adrenocorticotrophic hormone, gonadotrophic hormone, antidiuretic hormone, oxytocin, thyroxin, parathyroid hormone, epinephrine, norepinephrine, adrenal steroids, insulin, glucagon, testosterone, estrogen, progesterone, gonadotrophins, progesterone.

August, 1969   CMRI
Roanoke, Virginia

CONTENTS

SECTION I

CELL PHYSIOLOGY

An individual is, in essence, a collection of cells. Although the cells of the body are of various types and may have specific functions, there are certain properties shared by all cells. The general properties discussed in this section have been selected with regard to their utility in this physiology program.

1. Physiology is a study of the function of living systems. Living systems of concern to the physiologist range from entire organisms to parts of an organism such as a heart or kidney or a single cell. Thus a

   physiologist may choose to study living _____ at various levels of organization.

2. Three such levels of organization are the organ level, involving, for example, the heart, kidneys, or adrenal glands; the systemic level, concerned, for example, with the circulatory, renal, or endocrine

   _____ ; and the total structural level of organization.

   systems

3. Every living system depends, both for its structure and for its function, upon the nature of the cellular building blocks that compose it, whatever its level

   of _____.

   systems

1

4. Thus, we may consider a living _____ to be a population of component cells.

   organization

5. The branch of physiology that deals with the function and interactions of these cellular building blocks is called cell _____.

   system (organism)

6. The study of cell physiology concerns the relation between the _____ itself and the surroundings, called the cellular environment.

   physiology

7. Thus the fluid just outside of, but directly in contact with, the cell surface is called the cellular

   _____.

   cell

8. All fluids outside of the cells are referred to as

   extra _____ fluids.

   environment

9. The extracellular fluids of the body are classified as *interstitial fluids* (fluid lying in the spaces between cells), *plasma* (the fluid, noncellular part of the blood), and *special fluids* (such as those found in the central nervous system and gastrointestinal tract). The three types of extracellular fluids are

   interstitial, plasma, and _____ fluids.

   extracellular

10. Plasma refers to the fluid, non _____ part of the blood.

    special

11. The types of extracellular fluids are _____

    _____, and _____.

    noncellular

12. The interstitial fluid is in close contact with the cells of the body. Therefore, this fluid makes

    up the cells' _____.

    plasma
    interstitial, special

13. The total fluid volume in the body of a person weighing 150 to 160 pounds is about 40 liters. Of this total volume about 25 liters is intracellular

    fluid volume. The remaining _____ liters is

    _____ fluid volume.

environment

14. Thus the greater portion of the total fluid volume of the normal person is (extracellular/intracellular) fluid.

15
extracellular

15. You may recall that cell physiology is defined as a

    study of cell _____.

intracellular

16. One aspect of cell physiology is concerned with the

    relation between a cell and its _____.

function

17. The most general feature of cellular activity is the maintenance of a nonequilibrium relationship with the cellular environment. Injury and disease are disruptions of normal cellular activity. This means that the normal relationship with the cellular

    _____ is disrupted.

environment
(surroundings)

18. Remember that if a nonequilibrium relation with the cellular environment is the normal state, then

    the abnormal state would be _____
    with the environment.

environment

19. The nonequilibrium relation between the cell and its environment is evident in the differences in composition of the intracellular fluid and the interstitial

    or _____ fluid.

equilibrium

20. The following table shows the approximate concentrations of cellular and interstitial electrolytes, in mm/liter.

extracellular

3

Ion	Interstitial	Intracellular
Na^+	145	12
K^+	4	155
Cl^-	120	4
HCO_3^-	27	8
HPO_4^-	2	11
Mg^{+2}	2	30
SO_4^{-2}	0.5	1
Ca^{+2}	3	–

It may be seen from the table that the various elec-

trolyte concentrations within the _____ are generally quite different from the concentrations

_____ of the cell.

21. Refer to the table to complete the next few frames.
Compared to the intracellular fluid, sodium ion
(Na^+) is over twelve times (more/less) concentrated
in the interstitial fluid.

    cell
    outside

22. On the other hand, potassium ion (K^+) is about
forty times more concentrated (within/outside of)
the cell.

    more

23. Thus the nonequilibrium state between the cell and
its environment is demonstrated by these examples
of ion concentration differences inside and outside

   a _____ .

    within

24. The unequal distribution of materials is maintained
as long as the cell lives; therefore nonequilibrium is

   evidence that the cell is _____ .

    cell

25. When a cell dies, materials inside and outside of
the cell tend to equilibrate; that is, the cell ap-

   proaches a condition of _____

   with its _____ .

    alive (functioning)

26. The concepts of equilibrium and nonequilibrium
are illustrated by the following model:

    equilibrium
    environment

4

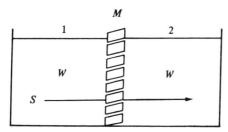

The model is a tank having two compartments, 1
and 2, separated by a membrane *M*. The tank is
filled with water *W*. Suppose that a substance *S*
were added to compartment 1 but not to compartment 2. *Initially then,* the concentration of substance *S* is (equal/unequal) on the two sides of the
membrane.

27. Now suppose that the membrane permits the pas-   unequal
    sage of substance *S*. The concentration of *S* will
    eventually become *equal* on the two sides of the
    membrane. The system will then have reached a

    state of _____ with respect to the
    distribution of substance *S*.

28. The living cell, however, is in a state of   equilibrium

    _____ with its environment.

29. One factor that *might* keep intracellular substances   nonequilibrium
    from reaching equilibrium with the cellular envi-
    ronment is the *lack of permeability* to these sub-

    stances of the cell wall or cell _____.

30. We have just considered the tendency of a sub-   membrane

    stance to reach _____ in a
    fluid system.

31. The phenomenon of *diffusion* is illustrated by this   equilibrium
    tendency of a substance in a fluid system to ap-

    proach _____.

5

32. *Diffusion* is the flow of a substance from a region of *higher* concentration to a region of *lower* concentration. In the model shown in Frame 26, which compartment, 1 or 2, initially had the higher concentration of substance *S*? Was the equilibration we observed an example of diffusion?

equilibrium
(equilibrate)

33. Diffusion refers to the flow of a *substance* from a

region of _____ concentration to a region of

_____ concentration of that substance.

compartment 1
yes

34. As the difference in concentration of a substance becomes smaller the rate of diffusion becomes slower. That means that if the difference in concentration of a substance between two compart-

ments is small, the rate of flow will be _____.

higher
lower

35. However, diffusion is usually faster through a membrane with a larger area than through one with a smaller area. Thus if the area of a membrane is decreased we would expect the diffusion rate to be (retarded/increased).

slow

36. The thickness of the membrane and the rate of diffusion are inversely related. Thus, an increase in the thickness would (increase/decrease) the rate of diffusion flow.

retarded

37. The rate of diffusion, dependent on several factors, is expressed by Fick's law:

decrease

$$F = \frac{DA(C_1 - C_2)}{X}$$

where   *F* is the flow
D is the diffusion coefficient
A is the area of the membrane through which flow occurs
X is the thickness of the membrane
$C_1 - C_2$ is the difference in concentration of the substance between compartment 1 and compartment 2.

Based on the relationships expressed by Fick's law, if the concentration difference is decreased, the rate of flow will (decrease/increase).

38. Increased thickness of the membrane will (decrease/increase) the flow.

decrease

39. Decreased area of the membrane through which a substance flows will (decrease/increase) the rate of diffusion.

decrease

40. To summarize, according to Fick's law, a substance diffuses from a _____ concentration to a _____ concentration until it reaches a state of _____ in which $C_1 = C_2$.

decrease

41. Sometimes differences in concentrations of substances inside and outside of the cell are due to a _____ of permeability (impermeability) of the cell membrane to these substances.

higher
lower
equilibrium

42. And, sometimes, there are unequal concentrations of a substance on either side of a membrane even though the membrane *is* _____ to the substance.

lack

43. One theory that explains (with respect to permeable materials) this nonequilibrium condition is called the pump theory. It is illustrated below.

permeable

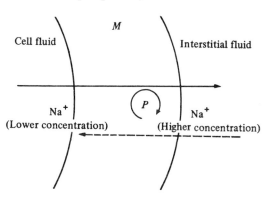

44. In this figure, *M* represents the cell membrane and *P* represents the pump mechanism. The concentration of Na^+ is *higher* on the interstitial side (*outside*) of the membrane. According to the definition of diffusion (Frame 32), in which direction would Na^+ tend to diffuse if unopposed?

45. In contrast, the sodium pump operates to move sodium (Na^+) from a region of _____ concentration to one of _____ concentration.

from outside to inside (from higher concentration to lower concentration)

46. Therefore the sodium pump acts opposite to the _____ of sodium from a region of _____ concentration to a region of _____ _____.

lower, higher

47. Any mechanism that moves a system away from equilibrium requires the utilization of cellular energy.

diffusion
higher
lower concentration

48. In an analogous fashion, pumping water uphill requires a source of _____. So, although the exact nature of the sodium _____ has not been determined, it would require an expenditure of _____.

49. Energy is the capacity to do work.

energy, pump, energy

50. Pumping water uphill or pumping Na^+ from a lower to a higher concentration is _____ and therefore requires a source of free _____. Free energy is that portion of the total energy which is actually available to do _____.

51. The free energy for the sodium pump is derived from the metabolism of food by the cell. The cell takes in food high in free energy and thus is able to perform its cellular work by utilizing some of this

_____ _____.

work
energy
work

52. The waste products of food metabolism, discarded by the cell, are (higher/lower) in free energy.

free energy

53. Although the exact mechanism by which the cell utilizes metabolic free _____ to operate the _____ pump is not known, ATP (adenosine triphosphate) is known to play a vital role.

lower

54. Adenosine triphosphate, or _____, is a high energy compound formed from ADP (adenosine diphosphate) by cellular _____.

energy
sodium

55. The free energy derived from food is usually not utilized immediately but is stored until needed as molecules of ATP, that is, _____

_____.

ATP
metabolism

56. Then, as energy is needed by the cell to perform its _____, molecules of ATP are *reconverted* to ADP with a release of _____ _____.

adenosine triphosphate

57. Although not equal, the individual concentrations of most substances inside and outside of the cell remain fairly constant. Thus, to maintain the concentrations of sodium inside and outside of the cell at a fairly constant level, the amount of Na^+ that is pumped out of the cell must be (more than/less than/equal to) the amount of Na^+ that diffuses back into the cell.

work, free energy

58. Let's quickly review. The Na^+ pump acts in an opposite direction to sodium _____.

equal to

9

59. To operate the Na⁺ pump, the cell reconverts
(ADP/ATP) to release the needed _____.

60. Thus the amount of Na⁺ in a cell remains
_____.

61. The term *sodium leak* refers to the flow or diffusion of Na⁺ *into* a cell. In the figure in Frame 43, the solid arrow indicates the direction in which

Na⁺ is moved by _____ _____. The dotted arrow indicates the direction in which Na⁺ leaks or

_____.

62. The pump-leak concept may also be applied to the distribution of potassium ion (K⁺). Refer to the table in Frame 20 to complete the next frame.

The pump moves K⁺ (into/out of) the cell and K⁺ leaks (into/out of) the cell.

63. It has been proposed that one pump mechanism may serve to move both Na⁺ and K⁺ across the cell membrane. This concept is illustrated in the figure below.

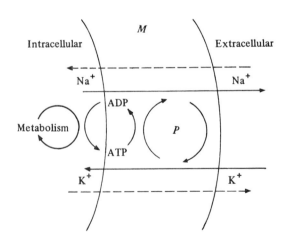

diffusion

ATP
energy

constant

the pump
diffuses

into
out of

In this figure the pump mechanism is shown coupled to ATP which in turn is coupled to cellular metabolism. The physical location and nature of the pump mechanism are matters of current investigation.

The proposed movement of a substance by a pump is called *active transport* since it involves the active expenditure of energy. This energy is derived from

ATP, which was synthesized from _____, using

free energy derived from _____.

64. Thus, cell metabolism provides the energy for the proposed movement of a substance by a pump,

which is called _____ _____.

ADP
metabolism

65. Free energy is released when _____ is reconverted

into _____.

active transport

66. Thus, active transport requires the energy derived

from _____.

ATP
ADP

67. Any interference with metabolism (e.g., poisoning, anoxia, starvation) will, in turn, cause a decrease in

_____ _____.

metabolism
or ATP

68. The leak of a substance is called "passive transport" because it does not depend on an expenditure of

cellular _____.

active transport
or ATP

69. When a cell ceases to function (dies) passive transport of materials proceeds unchecked by active transport. What would you expect to occur between the cell and its environment?

energy or ATP

70. Another theory of cellular distributions states that the unequal distribution of materials across the cell membrane occurs because of the movement of

metabolites across the _____.

The cell can be expected to approach a state of equilibrium with its environment

11

71. The major metabolites of most cells are glucose, oxygen, carbon dioxide, and water. Glucose and oxygen (anabalites) enter the cell and carbon dioxide and water (catabolites or products) leave the cell. The metabolites that enter the cell are

_____ and _____, and the metabolites that leave the cell are _____ _____ and _____.

Refer to the figure below to complete the next few frames.

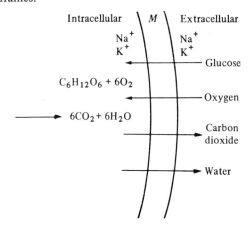

72. The theory states that the influx of metabolites (glucose and O_2) and the efflux of metabolites (CO_2 and H_2O) across the membrane interact with electrolytes (e.g., Na^+ and K^+) to prevent their diffusion toward an equilibrium distribution.

An analogy is in order. In the figure below consider how a constant flow of air will keep a suspended ping-pong ball from reaching its equilibrium position.

The degree of displacement of the ping-pong ball depends on the rate of flow of _____.

membrane

glucose, oxygen
carbon dioxide, water

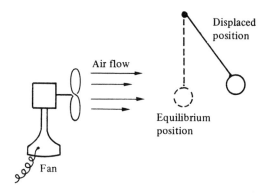

73. Similarly, the displacement of electrolytes from a condition of equal concentrations across the cell membrane depends on the rates of flow of

_____.

air

74. In this proposed theory for cellular distributions, the nonequilibrium concentration of electrolytes is maintained by the constant flow of _____.

metabolites

75. The rates of flow of these metabolites in turn depend on the rate of metabolism within the cell. Thus, if the metabolic rates are changed by the addition of certain drugs, it follows that the distributions of electrolytes will _____.

metabolites

76. Remember that the pump theory for explaining nonequilibrium distributions of electrolytes required a source of _____ _____.

change

77. This energy was said to come from the degradation of food, a process known as _____.

free energy

78. The cellular distribution theory just presented also requires a source of _____ _____ which is the product of _____.

metabolism

79. This theory is called the "interaction" theory due to the proposed interactions of the _____ and _____ involved.

free energy

metabolism

80. We have now considered two theories for a cellular function to explain the maintenance of

non _____ condition. Both required a source of _____ _____.

metabolites

electrolytes

81. You may rightly conclude that a system *not* coupled to a source of free energy will tend toward equilibrium. There are many paths a system may follow in approaching equilibrium. The particular path followed will depend on the concentrations of all constituents of the system and their relative permeabilities.

nonequilibrium

free energy

82. The next figure represents a two-phase system, phase 1 and phase 2. The phases are separated by a membrane *M*. (A phase is equivalent to a compartment.)

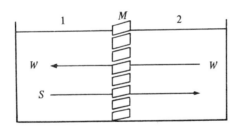

83. If the system contains only water *W*, we would not expect water to flow in either direction, since the concentration of water on both sides of the membrane would be _____.

84. If a substance *S* is added to phase 1, the concentration of *S* in phase 1 is (more/less) than its original value of zero; however, the concentration of *water* in phase 1 is now (more/less) than its original value.

equal

14

85. Thus, the addition of S dilutes the water in phase 1, and so the concentration of water is (increased/ decreased).

more
less

86. Concentration is an amount per unit volume. When S is dissolved in the water, it displaces some of this water from the unit volume. The *amount* of water in this unit volume becomes (more/less) and, consequently, the *concentration* of W becomes (greater/less).

decreased

87. Refer to the figure in Frame 82. Now, if the membrane M is equally permeable to W and S, water will diffuse to the (left/right), and S will diffuse to the (left/right).

less
less

88. In diffusion a substance moves from a region of

_____ concentration to a region of _____ concentration.

left
right

89. The flows of W and S will continue until an equilibrium is reached. In other words, W and S will

reach _____ concentrations throughout the system.

higher
lower

equal

NOTE: The following frames deal with a special case of diffusion called osmosis. Remember that in the general case of diffusion a substance tends to flow from a region of higher concentration to one of lower concentration. In osmosis, water flows from a higher concentration to a lower concentration of water, while the flow of solute is restricted by a membrane. Osmotic forces play an important part in the movement and distribution of water across cell membranes. The principles illustrated in this section will be utilized in later sections in the discussion of capillary water exchange, glomerular filtration, and body water balance.

Suppose the membrane of the system shown in the previous figure is semipermeable, that is, permeable to W, but not to S. Then, the only flow that can occur is (W/S) to the (right/left).

90. This system, which approaches equilibrium by the flow of water alone, has a membrane that is semipermeable.

W, left

15

91. *Osmosis* refers to diffusion restricted by a

semi _____ membrane.

92. The next figure shows another arrangement of a two-phase system.

semipermeable

W
1 S
2 W
(a)

P
W
1 S
2 W
(b)

The membrane separating the two phases is permeable to *W* but *im*permeable to *S*. Such a membrane

is said to be _____ .

93. Since the water concentration is lower in the phase containing *S*, water diffuses (into/out of) this phase.

semipermeable

94. As water moves into phase 1, the solution in phase 1 moves (up/down) the tube.

into

95. Remember that by virtue of its weight, the liquid in the tube will exert a force in a (downward/ upward) direction.

up

96. On the other hand, osmosis (movement of water) exerts a force in a(n) (downward/upward) direction.

downward

97. Movement of water (osmosis) will continue until

the system reaches a state of _____ .

upward

98. At equilibrium, the force driving water into phase 1 (due to the concentration difference of water, $C_1 - C_2$) and the force exerted by the weight of the

column of solution will be _____ .

equilibrium

16

99. Both forces are exerted on the total area of the

    _____.   equal

100. The weight of the column of water exerts a   membrane
     force. A force per unit area is a pressure. Thus,
     when the level of solution in the tube becomes
     constant, the pressure (P) exerted by the col-

     umn is equal and opposite to the _____ per

     unit _____ due to the concentration difference
     $C_1 - C_2$ of water across the membrane.

101. The force per unit area due to the concentration   force
     difference is called the osmotic pressure (π).   area
     Therefore, the system reaches equilibrium when
     the (area/pressure) of the column equals the

     _____ pressure.

102. The force per unit area on a membrane, due to the   pressure
     concentration difference of water, is the   osmotic

     _____ _____.

103. The *concentration of solute particles* in the solu-   osmotic pressure
     tion is one of the factors that determines the

     amount of _____ pressure.

104. One influence on osmotic pressure is the concen-   osmotic

     tration of _____ particles in the solution.

105. An increase in solute particle concentration will   solute
     decrease the water concentration and (increase/
     decrease) the osmotic pressure.

106. Another factor that determines osmotic pressure is   increase
     the *absolute temperature* of the solution. If os-
     motic pressure varies *directly* with temperature,
     how would you expect the pressure to change
     when the solution temperature is increased?

17

107. Thus, osmotic pressure varies directly with the

absolute _____ of the solution and

with _____ _____ concentration.

108. An increase in absolute temperature will (increase/
decrease) osmotic pressure.

109. Osmotic pressure will decrease with a *decrease* in

_____ _____ and a

decrease in _____ _____

_____.

110. The number of *osmols per liter* is one way of ex-

pressing the _____ of solute
particles.

111. One of the ways solute particle concentration is

expressed is in _____ per _____.

112. An osmol is a function of the molecular weight of
the solute. The molecular weight of a substance is
the sum of the atomic weights of the constituent
atoms of the molecule. For example, glucose is a
sugar molecule composed of carbon, hydrogen, and
oxygen atoms. The molecular weight of glucose is

therefore the sum of the weights of the ___, ___,

and ___ atoms present.

113. Notice that in glucose ($C_6H_{12}O_6$) there are 6 car-

bon, 12 hydrogen, and 6 _____ atoms.

114. The atomic weights of these elements are:

C = 12
H = 1
O = 16

If one carbon atom has a relative weight of 12,

then six carbons will weigh _____.

pressure is increased

temperature
solute particle

increase

absolute temperature
solute particle
concentration

concentration

osmols
liter

C (carbohydrate),
H (hydrogen),
O (oxygen)

oxygen

18

115. What is the molecular weight of the whole glucose molecule ($C_6H_{12}O_6$)?

72 (6 × 12)

116. The *gram molecular weight* of a compound is its molecular weight (glucose 180) expressed in terms of _____.

molecular weight 180

117. Therefore, the *gram* molecular weight of glucose is 180 _____.

grams

118. It is often convenient to express the concentration of dissolved substances as some number of gram molecular weights per liter of _____.

grams

119. The term *mole* is a shorter expression for gram _____ weight.

solution

120. Gram molecular weight and _____ are synonyms.

molecular

121. A *one* molar solution (1*M*) refers to *one* mole of solute in *one* liter of solution. One mole of glucose in one liter of solution makes up a one molar solution of glucose. How many moles of glucose are present in one liter of a 0.5*M* solution?

mole

122. And how many *grams* of glucose are there in 1 liter of a 0.5 molar solution?

0.5 moles

123. A solution of 1 molar glucose means 1 mole of glucose molecules or *particles* per liter of solution. But 1 mole of sodium chloride (NaCl) provides *more* than 1 mole of particles per liter.

$$\frac{180g}{mole} \times \frac{0.5\ moles}{liter} =$$
90 grams per liter

Acids, bases, and salts, you may recall, dissociate in solution as is shown by the following examples:

$$HCl \rightarrow H^+ + Cl^-$$
$$NaOH \rightarrow Na^+ + OH^-$$
$$NaCl \rightarrow Na^+ + Cl^-$$

124. Salts in solution dissociate almost completely into their component ions. One mole of NaCl, then,

provides almost ____ (how many?) moles of ions or particles.

125. Previously, when we talked about aqueous systems we saw that the addition of a substance to water causes the concentration of water to (increase/decrease).

2

126. This change in solvent (water) concentration is generally independent of the type of solute added. When particles of solute are added to a solution the solvent concentration is (increased/decreased) and the osmotic pressure is (increased/decreased).

decrease

127. Calculation of the osmotic pressure of a solution involves a C, or concentration term, which should be expressed as the number of osmols per

____.

decreased
increased

128. This solute concentration (C) is expressed as the

number of ____ ____ ____.

liter

129. In other words, osmolarity refers to the number of moles of solute particles per liter of solution. Thus, 1 mole of glucose (which does not dissociate) per

liter is ____ (how many?) osmolar (osM).

osmols per liter

130. But 1 mole of NaCl which dissociates into about 2

moles of ____ per liter becomes about

____ (how many?) osmolar.

1

131. According to the expression $MgCl_2 \rightarrow Mg^{+2} + 2Cl^-$, how many moles of particles does a mole of $MgCl_2$ provide in solution when it dissociates?

particles
2

132. Thus, 1 mole of $MgCl_2$ in a liter of water makes a

____ osM solution.

3

133. Absolute temperature is determined by adding 273 degrees to the temperature of the solution in degrees centigrade. How many degrees is 27°C expressed on the absolute scale?

3

134. Now let's see how we determine osmotic pressure. The approximate osmotic pressure of a solution can be calculated by the equation:

300

$$\pi = CRT$$

where C = the concentration of solute particles in the solution (osM/liter)
R = the gas constant (0.0821 liter atmospheres per degree per osmol) (liter atm/deg/osmol)
T = the absolute temperature (deg)
π, then, is given in atmospheres (atm).

135. Substitution of the given dimensional units for the symbols in the above equation looks like the following: Complete the equation (You may refer to Frame 134).

$$\pi = CRT$$
$$\pi = \frac{(osmols)}{(liter)} \frac{(\qquad)}{(deg\ osmol)} (\qquad)$$

136. Now, by using a form of dimensional analysis you can reduce the equation. Common units on the right side of the equation may be canceled to give the units of the answer. We have begun the analysis. Complete the cancelation and reduce the equation.

$\pi = \dfrac{(osmols)}{(liter)}$
$\dfrac{(liter\ atm)\ (deg)}{(deg\ osmol)}$

$$\pi = \frac{(osmols)}{(\cancel{liter})} \frac{(\cancel{liter}\ atm)}{(deg\ osmol)} (deg)$$

$$\pi = \underline{\hspace{5cm}}$$

NOTE: This method can be used to check your use of consistent units in physical equations.

137. Now calculate the osmotic pressure of a 2 molar glucose solution at 27°C.

Remember: glucose does not dissociate in water; therefore, a 2 molar glucose solution must equal a

_____ osM glucose.

Complete the problem. The correct response is given in the next frame.

$$\pi = \frac{(\text{osmols})}{(\text{liter})}$$
$$\frac{(\text{liter atm}) \, (\text{deg})}{(\text{deg osmol})}$$
$$\pi = \text{atmospheres (atm)}$$

138. The problem is: Calculate the osmotic pressure of a 2 molar glucose solution at 27°C. Here are the operations.

$$\pi = CRT$$
$$C = 2 \text{ osM}$$
$$R = 0.0821 \text{ (constant)}$$
$$T = 300° \, (27°C + 273°)$$
$$\pi = 2 \, (.0821) \, (300)$$
$$\pi = 49.5$$

In what units should we express the answer?

2

139. Now calculate π at 25°C for 0.3 moles of NaCl dissolved to make 1 liter of solution. Show your operations. (Hint: 0.3M NaCl = 0.6 osM NaCl)

atmospheres (atm)

See correct answer
in next frame

140. $C = 0.6$ $R = .0821$ $T = 298$
$$\pi = (0.6) \, (.0821) \, (298)$$
$$\pi = \text{about 14.7 atmospheres}$$

Although π may be expressed in atmospheres as above, it may also be expressed as millimeters of mercury (mm Hg). 1 atm = 760 mm Hg. What is the osmotic pressure of this solution expressed in millimeters of mercury?

22

141. A solution having the *same osmotic pressure* as a second solution is said to be *isosmotic* with respect to the second solution.

A solution with a greater osmotic pressure than another solution is *hyper*osmotic; a *hypo*ösmotic solution would have a (higher/lower) osmotic pressure than the reference solution.

(14.7 atm. X 760 mm Hg)
11,172 mm Hg

142. The preceding discussion dealt with the special case of diffusion called _____.

lower

143. Now let's conclude this section on cell physiology by relating these osmotic phenomena with the observable behavior of cells. All relations between the cell and its environment are mediated by the

cell_____.

osmosis

144. This membrane offers various degrees of resistance to the passage of different substances; it is especially permeable to water. Under comparable conditions the movement of water across the cell

_____ is much more rapid than the movement of sodium or potassium ions.

membrane

145. In this sense the cell membrane may be considered semipermeable; that is, the permeability to water is much (greater/less) than the permeability to ions.

membrane

146. In this osmotic system, the intracellular fluid is separated from the interstitial fluid by what may

be considered a _____ permeable membrane.

greater

147. Although the compositions of the intracellular and interstitial fluids are different, the calculated osmotic pressures—based on the total concentration of all solute *particles*—are very nearly equal in the two fluids. These fluids may be considered as

being_____ to each other.

semipermeable

23

148. A solution is said to be *isotonic* with respect to a
cell if the cell is placed in a solution and the cell
neither swells or shrinks. That is, the cell neither

    takes in water nor loses _____.

        isosmotic

149. If a cell swells in solution, the solution is (hypo-
tonic/hypertonic); if it shrinks, the solution is
(hypotonic/hypertonic).

        water

150. These definitions of tonicity are *functional* definitions—they are based on the behavior of a given
cell type in a given solution.

    Isosmotic and *isotonic* are not necessarily inter-
changeable terms. Isosmoticity is based on the

    _____ of the solution; iso-

    tonicity is based on the _____ of the cell.

        hypotonic
        hypertonic

151. A 0.3 osM NaCl solution is *isosmotic* with respect
to the intracellular fluid of red blood cells which

    would then also be about _____ osM.

        concentration
        behavior

152. Since red cells placed in this solution do not shrink
or swell for a given length of time, this isosmotic

    solution is also _____.

        0.3

153. Although a 0.3 cell osM urea solution is isosmotic
to normal red cells, red cells placed in such a solution swell and burst. Therefore the solution is not

    *iso*tonic, it is _____.

        isotonic

        hypotonic

NOTE: *The reason for the above behavior of the red cell despite the isosmotic
nature of the solution is based on the fact that the red cell membrane is highly
permeable to urea. The urea distributes rapidly across the membrane increasing
the total particle concentration within the cell. The cell fluid is now* hyperosmotic *with respect to the outside solution. Consequently water flows into the
cell causing it to swell and burst.*

154. The cell membrane is composed of proteins and
lipids arranged in layers.

24

155. The membrane is electrically polarized; that is, the surfaces of the membrane carry an electrical

_____ .

156. The membrane may contain *pores* through which materials pass into or out of the _____ .

charge

157. Material transport across the membrane may also occur by one or more carrier mechanisms. There is another means by which materials may cross the membrane in addition to movement through

_____ or via a _____ mechanism.

cell

158. Materials also may cross the cell membrane by dissolving *into* the membrane on one side and dissolving _____ of the membrane on the other side.

pores, carrier

159. For a substance to cross the cell membrane in this fashion it must be *soluble* in the material of the

_____ .

out

160. Since the cell membrane is partly lipid in nature, materials that are highly soluble in _____ generally can pass through the cell membrane quite easily.

membrane

161. Is the following statement true or false? Substances having very low lipid solubility generally pass freely across the cell membrane.

lipids

162. The degree of lipid *solubility* of a substance can be expressed by its relative _____ in oil and in water.

false

163. This solubility ratio is called an oil-water *partition coefficient.* The partition coefficient equals:

$$\frac{\text{solubility in?}}{\text{solubility in water}}$$

solubility

25

164. The higher a substance's partition coefficient, the more lipid soluble it is. Substance x has a high partition coefficient; substance y has a low partition coefficient. Which is expected to pass more freely through the cell membrane?

oil

165. A highly lipid soluble material is expected to have a relatively (high/low) diffusion coefficient.

x

166. Lipid solubility is an important factor in the rate of drug uptake by cells. A drug with a high lipid solubility generally crosses the cell membrane (quickly/slowly).

high (large)

167. Molecular size is another factor in the movement of a material across the _____ _____.

quickly

168. Larger molecules, in general, move more slowly than do _____ molecules.

cell membrane

169. A third factor affecting the movement of a substance across a cell membrane is electrical charge. Does the plasma membrane itself carry an electrical charge?

smaller

170. The movement of material across the cell membrane (which is itself charged) is related to the _____ charge on the particles of the material.

yes

171. An electrical charge on a particle, whether positive or _____ slows down the movement of this particle across the cell membrane.

electrical

172. Ions are charged particles. Do they move faster or more slowly than uncharged molecules?

negative

26

173. In summary, the permeability of a substance is re-   more slowly
     lated to three factors:

     its lipid _____,

     its molecular _____, and,

     its electrical _____.

174. Now let's review some of the concepts covered in   solubility
     this section. Physiology is a study of the   size
                                                          charge
     _____ of _____ systems.

175. A living system is a population of component   function, living

     _____.

176. Cell physiology is concerned with the functional   cells

     relationship between a _____ and its

     _____.

177. All fluid outside the cell is called _____   cell
     fluid.   environment

178. The fluid inside the cell is called _____   extracellular
     fluid.

179. Most of the fluid weight of the human body is   intracellular

     _____ fluid.

180. The most general feature of cellular activity is the   intracellular

     maintenance of a(n) _____ rela-

     tionship with the cellular _____.

181. Three types of extracellular fluid are _____,   nonequilibrium
                                                             environment
     _____, and _____ fluids.

182. As a cell dies, it approaches a state of   interstitial
                                                          plasma, special
     _____ with its _____.

27

183. Define diffusion.

184. The equation, $F = \dfrac{DA\,(C_1 - C_2)}{X}$ expresses _____ law.

185. The rate of diffusion varies directly with:

the _____ coefficient,

the _____ of the membrane, and

the difference in _____ of the substance between the two compartments.

186. The rate of diffusion varies *inversely* with the

_____ of the _____.

187. The energy for the pump mechanism comes from

the _____ _____ released when ATP is reconverted into ADP.

188. Metabolic energy is required for _____ transport.

189. _____ is synthesized from _____ using energy

derived from _____.

190. The "interaction" theory states that the influx of

_____ and _____ , and the efflux of

_____ and _____ prevent the diffusion of

_____ and _____ toward an equilibrium distribution across the cell membrane.

191. Define osmosis.

equilibrium
environment

The tendency of a substance to move from a region of higher concentration to a region of lower concentration.

Fick's

diffusion
area
concentration

thickness
membrane

free energy

active

ATP, ADP
metabolism

glucose, O_2
CO_2, water
Na^+, K^+

28

192. Osmotic pressure varies directly with the

_____ _____ of the solution and the concentration of _____

_____.

Diffusion restricted by a semipermeable membrane

193. The concentration of solute particles is expressed

in _____ ____ _____.

absolute temperature
solute particles

194. The word mole is a synonym for _____

_____ weight.

osmols per liter

195. One liter of a solution with one mole of solute is a

_____ solution.

gram
molecular

196. Acids, bases, and salts dissociate in solution.

NaOH (a base) would provide ___ particles upon dissociation.

molar or $1M$

197. Therefore 1 mole of NaOH introduced into a solution dissociates into ___ osmols.

2

198. How many moles of glucose are present in a liter of 5 molar solution?

2

199. How many grams of glucose are present in a liter of 0.8 molar solution? Remember that the gram molecular weight of glucose is 180 grams.

5

200. One mole of glucose per liter makes a ___ osmolar solution.

144 grams

201. One mole of NaCl per liter makes a ___ osmolar solution.

1

202. The gas constant may be expressed in _____

_____ per degree per osmol.

2

29

203. Write the formula for determining osmotic pressure.

204. π stands for _____ _____ and is expressed in terms of _____.

205. C stands for the _____ _____

_____.

R stands for the _____ _____.

T stands for the _____ _____.

206. To find the absolute temperature, add _____$^\circ$ to the temperature of the solution in degrees centigrade.

207. How many degrees is 44°C expressed on the absolute scale?

208. Two solutions that are isosmotic, that is, have the

same _____, also have the same

_____ pressure.

liter
atmospheres

$\pi = CRT$

osmotic pressure
atmospheres

solute particle
concentration
gas constant
absolute temperature

273°

317°

osmolarity
(osmotic concentration)
osmotic

This completes Section I on Cell Physiology. We recommend a short break before beginning Section II, Nerve-Muscle Physiology.

SECTION II

NERVE-MUSCLE PHYSIOLOGY

In this section we'll deal with some properties of two special cell types—nerve cells (neurons) and muscle cells (muscle fibers). These cell types have all the general properties we discussed in the previous section; in addition the muscle cell has the property of contraction. Both of these cell types have the property of conduction.

Therefore, a certain familiarity with some basic concepts of electrical circuits is essential to the understanding of the conduction properties of nerve and muscle cells.

1. This figure represents a simple electrical circuit.

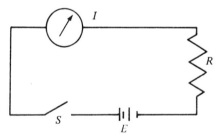

An ammeter measures the *current (I)*, R is a *resistance*, E is a source of *electromotive force*, and S is a switch to close the circuit.

2. The relation between E, I, and R is given by Ohm's law:

$$E = IR$$

or, in words, _____ _____

equals _____ times _____ .

3. If a current of 1 ampere (I) flows through a resistance of 1 ohm (R), (E) = 1 volt, which is called the

_____ _____ .

electromotive force
current, resistance

4. According to Ohm's law, the electromotive force needed to drive 2 amperes through a resistance of

3 ohms is ____ volts.

electromotive force

5. The next figure shows two electrodes (E_1 and E_2) immersed in a solution.

6

Voltmeter

E_1 Solution E_2

A metal immersed in an appropriate solution gives rise to an _electrical potential_, E_t. For example, copper wire in a copper sulfate solution gives rise to an

_____ _____ .

6. The electrical potential existing at an _electrode_ is

called an electrode _____ .

electrical potential

7. An electrode potential cannot be measured except

with reference to another _____

_____ .

potential

8. The potential of an _____ is related to the *concentration* of the solution in which it is immersed.

9. Two identical electrodes are hooked up (wired) to a voltmeter as shown in the above figure. The potentials of the two electrodes, E_1 and E_2, will be *equal* if the _____ of the solution is everywhere equal.

10. The two electrode potentials in this case, although _____ in magnitude, are opposite in sign with respect to the circuit.

11. The total electrical *potential* of the *circuit* (E_t) measured by the voltmeter, is the algebraic sum of all the _____ in the _____.

12. Translated into symbols this expression becomes:
    $$E_t = E_1 + E_2$$
    Now, provided that the concentration of solution is everywhere equal, E_1 and E_2 are _____ in magnitude but _____ in sign.

13. Expressed in symbols, this is
    $$E_t = E_1 + (-E_2).$$
    If $E_1 = E_2$, in magnitude

    Then, $E_t =$ _____

    Thus when the concentration of solution is everywhere _____, the total electromotive force in this system is _____.

33

14. In the next figure we have a situation similar to that of the last figure except that in this system there are two compartments separated by a membrane.

zero
equal
zero

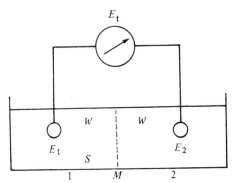

Identical electrodes are now put into the system in which the concentrations of a salt (*S*) (e.g., NaCl) are different on the two sides of the membrane.

15. The system will tend to approach equilibrium; that is, the _____ of salt will tend to become homogeneous throughout the system.

16. As discussed in the previous section, the two compartments can equilibrate by a flow of salt or water across the separating _____.

concentration

17. If the membrane is only slightly permeable to *S*, then *S* will move across the membrane only very _____.

membrane

18. Therefore, how fast the system approaches _____ will depend upon the resistance to diffusion offered by the _____.

slowly

19. In the system shown in the figure in Frame 14 there is another way in which equilibrium can be reached in addition to *salt and water movement* across the membrane.

The system can also approach ＿＿＿＿＿＿＿ via the external circuit connecting the two

＿＿＿＿＿＿＿ .

equilibrium
membrane

20. Because these electrodes are in solutions having different ＿＿＿＿＿＿＿ of salt, the potentials of E_1 and E_2 are (equal/not equal).

equilibrium
electrodes

21. Since E_1 does not equal E_2, the total electromotive force of the circuit $[E_1 + (-E_2)]$ is not equal to

zero. Going back to Ohm's law ($E = IR$ or $I = \underline{\ ?\ }$) we see that since there is an electromotive force when the circuit is closed, a current (I) will

flow. This movement of ＿＿＿＿＿ in the external part of the circuit is a flow of electrons.

concentrations
not equal

22. Current also moves in the solution, but this does *not* involve a flow of free electrons. Rather the current in solution consists of the movement of

ions, which are charged ＿＿＿＿＿＿＿ .

E/R
current

23. Resistance encountered at the membrane and in solution hampers the movement of ＿＿＿＿ .

particles

24. The flow of electrons through the external circuit (wire) is slowed by ＿＿＿＿＿＿＿ encountered in the wire.

ions

25. Thus equilibration of this system is retarded by two ＿＿＿＿＿＿＿ , one in the external *circuit* and one at the ＿＿＿＿＿＿＿ .

resistance

35

26. Since resistance R in the external circuit is very
    small, we see that the total electromotive force
    (E_t) is mainly a function of (is dependent on) E_1,

    E_2, and the _____ encountered at

    the _____.

    resistances
    membrane

27. There are many theories concerning the part played
    by the membrane in such a circuit. But it is generally

    held that a _____ to ionic flow oc-

    curs at the _____.

    resistance
    membrane

28. Other theories, rather than speaking of resistance
    at the membrane, attribute to the membrane an
    electromotive force of its own. The degree of
    polarization or charge orientation known to occur
    in the membrane is often considered a(n)

    _____ _____.

    resistance
    membrane

29. This polarization or charge orientation may result
    from the orientation of a charge pair (e.g., Na^+ and

    Cl^-) as it passes through the _____ or
    from a small increase in the distance between the
    members of the charge pair (charge separation) as

    they pass through the _____.

    electromotive force

30. A *membrane* exhibiting this charge orientation or
    polarization is said to exhibit an electrical *poten-
    tial.* Since the *membrane* exhibits this charge it is

    called a _____ _____.

    membrane
    membrane

31. The next figure is an elaboration of the previous
one in which the two phases are now separated by
a living membrane such as a section of frog skin.

membrane potential

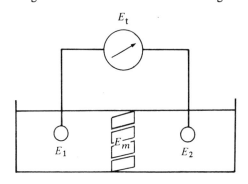

Under appropriate conditions an electrical

_____ can be measured in a circuit
such as that shown in this figure.

32. The total measured potential (E_t) is the sum of all

the _____ in the circuit.

potential

33. When E_1 and E_2 are equal in magnitude but opposite in sign, their effects cancel. Therefore, the
total measured potential must be due entirely to

the _____ .

potentials

34. Since the concentrations of Na^+ and K^+ inside and
outside the cell are so different, you can expect the

ion concentrations to influence the _____

_____ . In human cells measured membrane potentials are related to the concentrations
and permeabilities of Na^+ and K^+.

membrane

membrane potential

*NOTE: Although the figure varies somewhat with the method of measurement,
the measured value for the membrane of a resting nerve or muscle cell is about
−60 millivolts.*

35. The total measured potential is, in fact, dependent

on the differences in _____
of each ion on the two sides of the cell membrane.

37

36. The degree to which the cell membrane potential depends on each ion is related not only to the _____ in ionic concentrations but also to the _____ each ion meets in passing through the cell membrane.

concentrations

37. The membrane _____ is of great *functional* significance to nerve and muscle cells.

differences
resistance

38. The function of a nerve *fiber* is to conduct impulses from one point to another. A nerve _____ may conduct an impulse to another _____ _____ or directly to a muscle cell.

potential

39. The nerve *impulse* is an electrochemical change that is initiated at some point by a *stimulus* and moves along the nerve to another point. (See response area.)

The progression of an impulse along a _____ _____ occurs in a manner similar to the toppling of a row of dominoes.

fiber
nerve fiber

40. Although a single domino does not move far from its original position, it transmits the *impulse* it has received to the next in line. An impulse from one nerve fiber may serve as a(n) _____ to another nerve fiber which then carries the _____ to another point, or to a muscle cell, stimulating it to contract.

The original stimulus to a nerve may be mechanical, chemical, thermal or electrical!

nerve fiber

41. We have just considered a row of dominoes to represent a nerve _____. The first domino is pushed down by the stimulus and in turn topples the next one, and so on (the transfer of the impulse).

stimulus
impulse

42. Before another impulse can be transmitted by the row of dominoes, each domino must be returned to its original upright position. The analogous process following the transfer of an impulse in a _____ fiber is called *repolarization.*

fiber

38

43. The figure below illustrates the sequence of events that follows a stimulus to a nerve fiber.

nerve

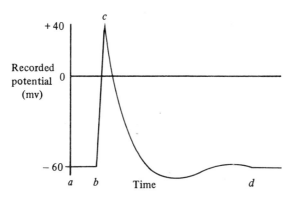

The initial part of the curve represents the normal or *resting* membrane _____ of a small segment of the nerve fiber. The normal resting potential of the nerve shown is _____ mv.

44. The section of nerve fiber where these membrane

_____ changes are occurring is called the *active site.*

potential
−60 mv (millivolts)

45. The rapid change of membrane potential (depolarization) that occurs at this segment of the nerve fiber (active site) after arrival of an impulse

amounts to about _____ mv.

potential

46. The spike in the curve is called the *action potential* of the nerve fiber. Notice on the graph that the potential rises quickly then drops back to below its original value and then returns to its original value,

called the _____ potential.

100 mv
(−60 mv to about
+40 mv)

47. The sudden change in membrane potential is related to an *increase* of permeability to sodium and to potassium. Consequently, the passive (leak) movements of these ions is (faster/slower).

resting

48. Na⁺ is about twelve times more concentrated

_____ the cell and K⁺ is about forty times

more concentrated _____ the cell. Therefore, how would you expect these ions to behave
when at the initiation of a spike potential it sud-
denly becomes much easier for them to traverse
the membrane?

The rates of these ion movements are *not* equal, *do
not* involve large quantities, and *do not* continue to
move for long periods of time.

faster

49. The *recovery* period (repolarization) involves a return to the original Na⁺ and K⁺ permeabilities of
the membrane and the restoration of the original
ionic concentration levels. Just as energy is required to set up a domino that has fallen, the recov-

ery process in a nerve requires a source of _____.

outside
inside
Na⁺ would move into
  cell
K⁺ would move out of
  cell

50. During its spike or action _____ the
active site of a nerve fiber is *absolutely refractory*—
that is, inexcitable.

energy

51. The *absolute refractory* period is followed by a
period during which only a strong stimulus can excite the nerve fiber. This is known as a partial

_____ period.

potential

52. The durations of the _____ periods
vary with the type of nerve fiber. For a large

_____ fiber this duration is about 1 millisecond (.001 sec). If recovery for each impulse in a
given nerve fiber takes 1 millisecond, what is the
maximum number of impulses that this nerve can
carry per second?

refractory

53. The active state of the nerve fiber is passed from
one *segment* of the nerve fiber to the next segment
by a circular flow of electric current, that is, a flow

of _____.

refractory
nerve
1000

40

54. The length of each segment depends on the insula-
tive properties of the myelin sheath surrounding the

    nerve _____ .

    ions

55. The indentations of the myelin sheath are called
nodes of Ranvier. Conduction from one node of

    _____ to the next is called saltatory con-
duction.

    fiber

    Ranvier

*NOTE: If a stimulus is applied to the center of a nerve fiber, saltatory conduc-
tion will proceed in both directions to each end of the fiber. Normally, however,
the stimulus is given at one end of the fiber and the impulse proceeds in one
direction.*

56. Nerve fibers vary in size and in velocity of impulse
conduction. There are three main groups—*A, B,*
and *C.*

    Group *A* nerve _____ are highly myelinated
and are found in nerve bundles serving *sensory* and
motor functions. Fibers of this group are the fastest conductors.

57. Group *B* fibers conduct _____ more
slowly than group *A* fibers and constitute the preganglionic autonomic fibers.

    fibers

58. Group *C* fibers are the slowest conductors of

    _____. These are the so-called nonmye-
    linated* fibers.

    impulses

59. The types of fibers and average conduction veloci-
    ties (meters per second) are given below:

Type	Velocity
A	5 m/sec to 120 m/sec
B	4 m/sec
C	1 m/sec to 3 m/sec

All nerve fibers act on the *all-or-none principle.*
That is, they never carry only part of an impulse
but transmit either a complete impulse or nothing
at all. (Could a domino, for example, transmit
only part of an impulse?)

impulses

60. The *magnitude* of a spike *potential,* therefore, de-
    pends only on the state of the nerve fiber at the
    active site and not on the magnitude of the stimu-

    lus causing the spike _____. For exam-
    ple, if the *stimulus* is more than adequate, still only
    a normal spike potential is produced. But an in-

    adequate _____ will not produce an

    action _____.

61. To sum up the all-or-none principle of impulse
    conduction we say that, given an adequate

    _____ the spike potential is independent

    of the *magnitude* of the _____.

    potential
    stimulus
    potential

---

*It has been found that all fibers have some degree of
myelination. The term "nonmyelinated," however, is
still used to describe those fibers having a very little
myelination.

62. Since the _____ of every spike poten-

tial is independent of the _____ strength
(as long as it is adequate), the only way a nerve
fiber can convey a message is through changes in
the number of impulses transmitted in a given time.

stimulus
stimulus

63. Consider a muscle that receives impulses from

many nerve _____. Although all individual
impulses are similar, the *total stimulus* to the mus-

cle will vary with the number of _____
received during a given time.

magnitude
stimulus

64. A series of _____ of increasing intensity
applied to a *group* of nerve fibers (a nerve trunk)
can produce a graded response of muscle contraction.

fibers
impulses

65. Although each fiber of the group obeys the _____

or _____ principle, each fiber may nevertheless
have a different *threshold* for excitation.

stimuli

66. As more fibers are excited by the increasing intensity of the applied stimulus, the total stimulus to
the muscle increases in magnitude, giving rise to
a(n) (increased/decreased) response of the muscle.

all
none

67. For a given nerve fiber, the effectiveness of an
electrical stimulus to the fiber depends on the
strength of the current and the time over which
this current is applied. If a weak current requires a
long time to initiate a *response* by a nerve, a strong
current will require (more/less) time to initiate the

same _____.

increased

68. No matter how strong a stimulus is, if it is applied

to the nerve for an *in*sufficient time, *no* _____
will be initiated.

less
response

69. If the current (stimulus) is too small, no _____ will occur however long the current is applied. This relation is illustrated by the strength-duration curve shown below.

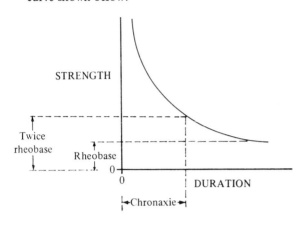

response

70. The minimum current strength needed to excite a given fiber is called *rheobase*.

response

71. The time necessary to cause excitation using a current strength of twice rheobase is called *chronaxie*. This time value, which provides a useful clinical index of nerve excitability and is used to characterize various diseased states of the nerve, is called

_____.

72. The time necessary to cause excitation using a current strength of twice _____ is called

_____.

chronaxie

73. Let's quickly review. Write the equation expressing Ohm's law.

rheobase
chronaxie

74. What does this equation mean?

$E = IR$

75. Two electrodes immersed in a solution with the concentration everywhere equal have potentials

that are _____ in magnitude and _____ in sign.

Electromotive force equals current times resistance

44

76. The total electrical potential of a circuit is equal to the algebraic sum of all the _____ in the _____.

equal, opposite

77. A two-compartment electrolyte system with appropriately connected electrodes can approach equilibrium by a flow of _____ through a membrane and by a flow of _____ through an external circuit.

potentials
circuit

78. The equilibration of this system is hindered by _____ in the _____, at the _____ and in the _____.

ions
electrons

79. One theory concerning the role of the membrane in the circuit states that a _____ to ionic flow occurs at the membrane.

resistances, wire, membrane, solutions

80. Another theory states that the membrane has its own source of _____ _____.

resistance

81. The measured value of the nerve membrane potential is about _____ mv.

electromotive force

82. Membrane potential is related to the concentrations of _____ inside and outside of the cell as well as to the _____ the _____ meet in passing through the _____.

−60 mv

83. A nerve fiber may conduct an _____ to a _____ _____ or to _____ cells.

ions
resistance, ions
membrane

84. An adequate stimulus brings about an electrochemical change in a nerve fiber called _____.

impulse
nerve fiber, muscle

45

85. A graph of the sequence of impulse conduction shows a *resting* phase, an *action* potential, and finally _____.

depolarization

86. The arrival of an impulse to a point on the nerve fiber brings about a total change of potential at that point of about _____ mv.

recovery
(repolarization)

87. The change in membrane potential is related to an increase in permeability to _____ and ____ ions.

100 mv
(−60 to +40)

88. During its spike potential, the nerve fiber is _____ refractory.

Na$^+$, K$^+$

89. This period is followed by a _____ _____ period.

absolutely

90. The durations of the _____ periods vary with the type of nerve fiber. For large fibers it is about _____.

partially
refractory

91. Conduction from one node of Ranvier to the next is called saltatory conduction.

refractory
1 m/sec

92. If a stimulus is applied to the center of a nerve fiber, _____ conduction will proceed in _____ directions to each end of the fiber.

93. Nerve fibers are classified according to velocity of _____ conduction.

saltatory
both

94. Group *A* nerve fibers are _____ myelinated and are involved in nerve bundles serving _____ and _____ functions.

impulse

highly
sensory
motor

95. Arrange the fiber groups in order of decreasing speed of conduction of impulses.

46

96. The fibers that are called nonmyelinated are group _____ fibers.

    A, B, C

97. All three groups of fibers act in accordance with the ____-_____-_____principle.

    C

98. The magnitude of the spike potential (is/is not) influenced by the magnitude of the stimulus if the stimulus is adequate.

    all-or-none

99. Since the _____ of spike potentials is independent of the strength of an adequate stimulus, the only way a nerve fiber can convey a different message is through a change in the number of _____ transmitted in a given _____.

    is not

100. A graded series of electrical stimuli applied to a nerve trunk can produce a graded _____ in a muscle.

    magnitude
    impulses, time

101. Each nerve fiber in the nerve trunk may have a different _____ for excitation.

    response

102. The effectiveness of an electrical stimulus to a nerve fiber is a function of the _____ of the current and the _____ over which it is applied.

    threshold

103. Rheobase is the term used to indicate the minimum current strength needed to _____ a fiber.

    strength
    time

104. Chronaxie is the term that indicates the period of time necessary for excitation to occur with a current _____ _____.

    excite

105. The insulator surrounding the nerve is called the _____ _____.

    twice rheobase

47

106. Another name for spike potential is ——————— potential.

107. The section of nerve fiber where changes in membrane potential are occurring is called the ———————

———————.

108. An *axon* is the long part of a nerve cell that carries impulses from the body of the nerve cell to the body of another nerve cell or to a *muscle cell.*

Every nerve cell has at least one ————————. Some axons are four or more feet long.

109. The function of nerve impulses is to alter the behavior of the cell which receives that ————————. What change might take place in a muscle cell which has received an impulse at its motor end plate?

110. The place where an axon meets a muscle cell is called a *motor end plate.*

111. In the figure below you see a diagram of a motor end plate.

Notice that the insulating material (myelin sheath) is not present where the axon meets the ———————— cell.

112. When an impulse reaches the flattened end of the
_____, *acetylcholine* (ACh) is released by the
axon into the nerve-muscle space, which brings
about a change in the _____ cell.

muscle

113. Acetylcholine acts to increase the *membrane* potential of the muscle cell _____.

axon
muscle

114. You'll recall that the normal cell membrane has an
electrical charge. This is known as the cell's

_____ _____.

membrane

115. The potential that is generated at the end plate is
called the *end plate* _____.

membrane potential

116. When the membrane potential of the muscle cell in
the region of the nerve axon (the endplate potential) reaches a critical magnitude, that is, when
enough acetylcholine reaches the muscle cell

_____, an action potential is induced at
the end plate.

potential

117. Thus, the attachment of acetylcholine to the membrane at the end plate leads to an increase in the
membrane _____ at this site.

membrane

118. This increase in _____ _____
at this site results in *depolarization* (reversal of
normal polarity) of the membrane.

potential

119. If the depolarization is sufficient, the result is a
muscle action potential propagated over the muscle
cell. This is similar to the nerve action _____.

membrane potential

120. The muscle _____ _____ moves
over the surface of the muscle cell causing the muscle cell to _____.

potential

121. Contraction results from depolarization of the muscle cell _____.

action potential
contract

122. The motor nerve releases _____ when stimulated by one or more nerve action _____.

membrane

123. Since *depolarization* is necessary for each contraction of the muscle cell, before another contraction can take place, the muscle cell membrane must be _____. (Can a domino be knocked over twice without being reset after it first falls?)

acetylcholine
potentials

124. If the acetylcholine released at the motor end plate were not promptly removed or destroyed, the muscle cell membrane would remain depolarized and the muscle could not be made to _____ again.

repolarized

125. However, an enzyme called *cholinesterase* is present at the nerve-muscle junction to facilitate the breakdown of acetylcholine into its components, acetate and choline. The removal of ACh by cholinesterase permits the muscle cell membrane to _____.

contract

126. Thus, by interference with the production or release of ACh at the motor end plate or by interference with the activity of cholinesterase, an impulse from a _____ cell to a _____ cell can be _____.

repolarize

127. Interference with the activity of cholinesterase would prevent repeated transmissions of impulses because ACh would remain at the end plate junction and the _____ would keep the membrane in a state of depolarization.

nerve, muscle
blocked

50

128. ACh release is favored by the presence of calcium ions and antagonized by magnesium _____.

muscle

129. Nerve-muscle impulse transmission is blocked by a drug called *curare.* Curare is sometimes used during surgery to relax _____.

ions

130. A single muscle is composed of many muscle cells or *fibers.* Each _____ is bounded by a cell membrane.

muscles

131. Each fiber is in turn composed of many *fibrils* grouped in bundles. Each _____ in turn consists of two types of myofilaments. Some are thick filaments and some are thin.

fiber (cell)

132. The thick and thin _____ are all parallel to each other. The thick filaments (myosin) are sandwiched between the thin filaments as shown below.

fibril

THICK AND THIN MYOFILAMENTS OF A FIBRIL

Sarcomere

133. The groups of thick _____ give the appearance of dark bands perpendicular to the direction of contraction. These dark bands are called the "A" bands of the muscle.

filaments

51

134. The lighter perpendicular bands are the *"I"* bands of the muscle. The striated appearance of voluntary muscle is due to the ____ bands and the ____ bands.

filaments

135. Refer to the diagram in Frame 132. The space between two *Z* lines in the diagram is called a

_____ and consists of an *A* band and parts of two *I* bands.

A, I

136. If each sarcomere were to shorten, the whole muscle would _____.

sarcomere

137. During contraction the thick and the thin filaments slide past one another or "telescope." Thus, contraction of the whole muscle is the result of shortening the _____.

contract (shorten)

138. Shortening of a _____ is initiated by an abrupt change in the local membrane potential (i.e., the muscle action potential).

sarcomeres

139. The contraction process is thought to be related to the making and breaking of chemical bonds between filaments in the _____.

sarcomere

140. The energy source for these reactions, and hence for muscle _____ itself, is the high-energy molecule ATP.

sarcomere

141. Any drug that interferes with the metabolic process leading to ATP formation eventually leads to a disturbance of muscle _____.

contraction

142. Again it's time to review what you've covered. The long part of a nerve cell that carries impulses from the body of the nerve cell to a muscle cell is the _____.

contraction

143. The insulator surrounding a nerve is the _____ sheath.

axon

144. The myelin sheath is not present at the _____ _____ _____ region.

myelin

145. When an impulse reaches the motor end plate region a chemical known as _____ is released by the nerve.

motor
end plate

146. This chemical increases the _____ _____ of the muscle cell at that site.

acetylcholine

147. When enough acetylcholine reaches the cell membrane, the membrane potential increases and _____ occurs.

membrane
potential

148. The potential generated at the end plate is called the _____ _____ _____ .

depolarization

149. A muscle action potential is similar to a _____ action potential.

end plate potential

150. After a muscle cell membrane has been depolarized and contraction has occurred, it must be _____ and then _____ again before another contraction can take place.

nerve

151. The enzyme _____ breaks down _____ into its components _____ and _____ .

repolarized
depolarized

152. ACh release is favored by the presence of _____ ions and antagonized by _____ ions.

cholinesterase
acetylcholine
acetate, choline

153. Nerve-muscle impulse transmission is blocked by _____ .

calcium, magnesium

154. A muscle is composed of many fibers, each of which is bounded by a _____ _____.

155. A fiber is composed of _____ grouped in bundles.

156. A fibril is made up of _____.

157. The thick filaments, _____, are sandwiched between _____ filaments.

158. The filaments appear as bands (*A* and *I*) perpendicular to the direction of _____.

159. When the sarcomeres shorten, the muscle _____.

160. Shortening of the sarcomere occurs following the spread of the muscle action _____ over the muscle cell.

161. The energy for contraction comes from _____.

162. The making and breaking of chemical bonds between the filaments in the sarcomeres is thought to account for _____ _____.

163. The contraction of a single sarcomere is too weak to make a whole _____ contract.

164. Therefore, shortening of the _____ of many *muscle fibers* at once is necessary to form a useful contraction.

165. *Maximum* muscle exertion would be achieved only when all the sarcomeres within _____ muscle fibers contract together.

curare

cell membrane

fibrils

filaments

myosin
thin

contraction

contracts

potential

ATP

muscle contraction

muscle

sarcomeres

166. The part of a nerve cell that carries the impulse to muscle fibers is the nerve _____.

all

167. One nerve axon may transmit impulses to a few or several hundred muscle fibers through branches of the same nerve _____.

axon

168. The stimulus transmitted by a _____ axon causes a twitch of each muscle fiber associated with that axon.

axon

169. The nerve cell body, the nerve axon, and all the _____ fibers that receive stimuli from this axon altogether are called a *motor unit*.

nerve

170. The nerve cell body (*a*), the nerve axon (*b*), and the muscle fibers stimulated by this axon (*c*) compose a _____ _____.

muscle

171. Name the parts of a motor unit.

motor unit

Motor end plate

Spinal cord

(*b*) Axon

(*c*) Muscle fibers .

(*a*) Cell body

172. Let's consider the contraction process in a little more detail. First we're going to focus our attention on the *anatomy* of the muscle fiber. The functional unit of the fiber (the parts whose shortening are actually responsible for whole muscle contraction) we have already called the _____.

1. nerve cell body
2. nerve axon
3. muscle fiber stimulated by this axon

173. *Actin* filaments and *myosin* filaments are located within the sarcomeres of the muscle _____.

sarcomeres

55

174. Actin and myosin filaments combine during con-
     traction to form actomyosin.   fibers

175. Energy to form actomyosin is supplied in chemical
     form by the high-energy molecule adenosine tri-

     phosphate, or _____.

176. Calcium ions must also be present in addition to   ATP

     the energy-rich _____.

177. The molecule ATP supplies the energy to form   ATP
     actomyosin, which is necessary for muscular

     _____. But for contraction to

     occur, there must also be a presence of _____
     ions.

178. If a muscle's length changes during a contraction,   contraction
     the contraction is called isotonic. A *change* in   calcium

     muscle length characterizes an _____
     contraction.

179. Isotonic contraction is said to have occurred when   isotonic

     the length of a muscle _____.

180. Muscle contraction may also be static (isometric).   changes
     In this case, the tension of the entire muscle in-

     creases but its _____ remains constant.

181. Muscle contraction characterized by an increase in   length
     muscle tension and no change in length is called

     isometric _____.

182. An increase in muscle tension at constant length is   contraction
     called _____ contraction; if muscle

     length changes it is an _____ contraction.

183. There is an optimum length at which the muscle can develop its greatest force, that is, develop its greatest _____.

isometric
isotonic

184. The optimum length for the production of maximum force is approximately the resting (normal) length of the muscle in its usual position in the body.

tension

185. Since the total force or tension developed is the sum of all the tensions developed by the individual fibers, the concerted efforts of *how many* fibers are needed for *maximum* tension of the muscle?

186. Because a single nerve axon usually stimulates the fibers of only a small part of a muscle, to excite *all* the muscle fibers, (few/many) nerve axons must be stimulated.

all of them

187. The number of muscle fibers stimulated to contract determines the degree of _____ of the whole muscle.

many

188. One impulse from a nerve fiber leads to the contraction of a certain number of _____ _____.

contraction

189. How much muscle contraction or tension would result from the stimulation of half of the muscle's fibers (relative to maximum tension)?

muscle fibers

190. The *contraction phase* of a muscle fiber lasts only a short time and is followed by a *relaxation phase.*

Only rarely would all motor _____ contract at the same time.

half maximum
tension

191. Usually some motor units are in the contraction phase, while other motor units are in the _____ _____.

units

192. A muscle can maintain a state of sustained contraction for a relatively long time because the individual _____ units alternate between

_____ and _____ phases.

relaxation phase

193. Neuromuscular diseases may be described in terms of the motor unit. So let's look more closely at this important unit. The nerve cell body of a

motor unit is located in the _____ cord.

motor
contraction
relaxation

194. The nerve cell axon leads from the _____

_____ to the muscle it serves.

spinal

195. Destruction of either the nerve cell _____ or the

nerve cell _____ results in a loss of function of the associated muscle fibers.

spinal
cord

196. If a sufficient number of motor units are destroyed,

the function of the entire _____ may be lost.

body
axon

197. When a muscle loses its nerve connections for any reason, two things generally follow. First, the entire muscle becomes increasingly sensitive to acetylcholine and related drugs. Second, after prolonged disuse the muscle will decrease in size. The entire muscle becomes increasingly sensitive to

_____ and related drugs.

muscle

198. After prolonged disuse the muscle will _____ in size (atrophy).

acetylcholine

199. *Myasthenia gravis* is a disease characterized by extreme muscle fatigue. The disease affects the region between the nerve and the muscle, which is known

as the _____ _____ plate.

decrease

200. Skeletal muscle is normally stimulated by the chemical _____ at the end-plate. Thus, one reason for fatigue may be insufficient release of the chemical _____.

motor end

201. A second explanation of myasthenia gravis could be too rapid a destruction of acetylcholine at the end plate by (too much/too little) acetylcholinesterase.

acetylcholine
acetylcholine

202. A third possible cause is a(n) (increase/decrease) in muscle sensitivity to acetylcholine.

too much

203. If excess acetylcholinesterase at the end plate is the cause, what would be the effect of administering an anticholinesterase?

decrease

204. Other muscular disorders (e.g., progressive muscular dystrophy) involve destruction of the contractile mechanisms of the _____ fibers.

a possible return to normal nerve-muscle impulse transmission

205. If a graded stimulus is applied to a nerve (containing the axons of many motor units) a graded response is shown by the muscle.

muscle

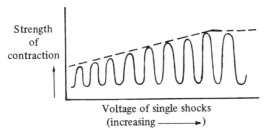

Voltage of single shocks
(increasing ——►)

In this figure the strength of a muscle's contraction reaches a (maximum/minimum) as the voltage applied to the nerve trunk is increased to a certain point.

206. At this maximal stimulus, how many motor units of the nerve-muscle preparation are responding to the stimulus? (most/all)

maximum

59

207. Remember that *each* motor unit of the preparation either responds or does not respond. What principle or law does this illustrate?

all

208. The number of units that respond to a given stimulus depends on the _____ of that stimulus.

all-or-none law

209. A supramaximal stimulus to the nerve trunk will elicit a muscle response (greater/no greater) than a maximal stimulus would elicit.

strength (magnitude)

210. There is, however, a variable in muscle contraction in addition to the stimulus strength. This is the time between stimuli. If maximal stimuli are given to the nerve such that the interval between successive stimuli is very short, the muscle will show an increased tension over that caused by a single maximal stimulus.

no greater

211. To elicit this effect, the time between _____ can be no shorter than the absolute refractory periods of the motor units.

212. The effect of an increased *rate* of stimulation is illustrated below:

stimuli

This summation of response to high-frequency _____ occurs because the contractile mechanism does not have _____ to fully relax between stimuli.

60

213. Tetanus (or tetany) is a neuromuscular disorder that may result from a low calcium level in the blood (hypocalcemia). The toxin, or poison, of a certain bacillus may also cause the neuromuscular

disorder known as _____.

stimulation
time

214. The frequency of nerve stimulation necessary to produce tetanus of a muscle varies with the muscle. About 100 stimuli per second are necessary to *tetanize* the biceps muscle, and a frequency of 30 stimuli per second to the soleus muscle will cause

_____.

tetanus

215. There are three types of muscle: striated (voluntary) muscle, smooth (involuntary) muscle, and cardiac muscle. In previous frames we discussed striated muscle (biceps, triceps, and other skeletal muscles),

which are also known as _____ muscles.

tetanus (tetany)

216. Smooth muscle is located in blood vessel walls and the organs of the body (such as the stomach, spleen, and bladder). This type of muscle is also

known as _____ muscle.

voluntary

217. Blood vessel walls and body organs contain

_____ or _____ muscle.

involuntary

218. Do you remember that the contraction process of *striated* muscle involves the muscle proteins or filaments, actin and myosin?

The contraction process of *smooth* muscle is be-

lieved to be the same as that of _____.
muscle.

smooth, involuntary

219. Smooth muscle contraction, then, involves the

muscle proteins _____ and _____ .

Do you?
striated

220. The contraction of smooth muscle, however, is slower and more prolonged than the contraction of striated muscle.

actin, myosin

61

221. Compared to striated muscle, smooth muscle contraction is (faster/slower) and lasts for a (longer/shorter) period of time.

222. As in striated muscle, smooth muscle contraction is initiated by changes in the muscle membrane

_____.

slower
longer

223. Nerve impulses to the muscle may bring about membrane potential changes that initiate smooth

_____ _____.

potential

224. But *local changes* in smooth muscle membrane potentials may occur spontaneously, and thus lead to

muscle _____.

muscle contraction

225. For example, stretching smooth muscle can change

the local membrane _____ and thus lead to contraction of the muscle.

contraction

226. A certain level of sustained contraction is exhibited by all muscle. This state of the muscle is called tone. Sustained contraction by smooth muscle at

a certain level is called _____.

potential

227. In addition to tone, smooth muscle may show rhythmic contractions related to spontaneous local

changes of the _____ _____.

tone

228. Smooth muscle is generally innervated by *autonomic* (sympathetic and parasympathetic) nerve fibers. These are the nerves that act to change the degree of muscle tone and change the rate of rhythmic contraction of _____.

membrane potential

229. Now let's look at another type of muscle. Cardiac

muscle (making up the walls of the _____) is

functionally similar to _____ muscle.

smooth
muscle

62

230. The contraction mechanism of each muscle type

(_____, _____, and _____) are thought to be the same.

231. A cell body and an axon make up the nerve cell, which is also called a neuron.

232. A synapse is the junction between two nerve cells,

that is, two _____.

233. Nerve impulses may pass in one direction only

across the _____.

234. Thus, impulses pass from the terminal knobs (pre-synaptic terminals) of one neuron to the cell body (or cell body projections—dendrites) of the successive _____.

235. Each cell body receives impulses from the terminal

_____ of many other neurons.

236. In other words, cell bodies have multiple synapses. This is illustrated in the following figure.

heart
smooth (involuntary)

striated, smooth
cardiac

neurons

synapse

neuron

knobs

Terminal knob

Myelin sheath

Cell body

An impulse arriving over a presynaptic neuron

causes the _____ knobs associated with that neuron to release a *transmitter substance.*

237. The transmitter substance may be an excitatory chemical or an inhibitory chemical. Suppose an excitatory transmitter substance *lowers* the membrane potential of the postsynaptic cell body. Which kind of chemical transmitter *increases* the membrane potential, thus making the cell body less excitable?

terminal

inhibitory

NOTE: The excitatory transmitter substance at synapses in the autonomic ganglia is acetylcholine. It is probable that acetylcholine is also the excitatory transmitter in CNS synapses, although it is possible that different types of excitatory trans-mitters—norepinephrine, 5-hydroxytryptamine, etc.—are secreted in different synapses. The nature of the inhibitory transmitter is not known, although some evidence indicates that gamma aminobutyric acid may be involved.

238. The excitatory transmitter reduces the membrane potential of the cell _____.

239. This reduced *potential* is called the _____ postsynaptic potential of EPSP.

body

240. If the EPSP is large enough (i.e., rises above a threshold value), an *action potential* will be initiated in the postsynaptic _____.

excitatory

241. The EPSP of a cell body can be raised to a _____ value by the combined action of many synapses.

neuron (cell body)

242. If the EPSP is maintained at a fairly high level (but still below threshold) by the continued action of many _____, the neuron is said to be facilitated. Is a facilitated neuron more easily excited than normal?

threshold

243. Additional presynaptic discharges can more easily induce an action potential in a neuron that has already been _____.

synapses
yes

244. The release of an inhibitory transmitter substance
at a _____ increases the membrane
_____ of the cell body.

245. Therefore, the increased membrane potential makes
the cell (more/less) excitable.

246. So, whether or not a cell body initiates an action
_____ depends on the overall effect of
excitatory and inhibitory substances released at its
surface by the many _____.

247. An impulse travels very rapidly over a nerve fiber
but much more slowly through a _____.

248. This slowing down is called synaptic delay. When
presynaptic terminals are repetitively stimulated at
a rapid rate, the postsynaptic _____
transmits fewer and fewer impulses.

249. *Synaptic fatigue* is the term used to describe this
slowdown in transmission of _____.

250. Synaptic _____ is presumed to be due to
the exhaustion of transmitter substance.

251. The remainder of the frames in this section constitute the final review.

252. Ohm's law describes the relations of resistance,
electromotive force, and _____.

253. The magnitude of an electrode potential is related
to the _____ of a solution.

254. The arrival of an impulse at a point on a nerve fiber
initiates a rapid electrochemical change termed the
_____ _____.

facilitated

synapse
potential

less

potential
synapses

synapse

neuron

impulses

fatigue

current

concentration

65

255. The recovery period following nerve impulse transmission requires _____.

action potential (spike)

256. Nerve impulses move along a fiber by _____ conduction.

energy

257. The least stimulus strength that can excite a nerve fiber is called _____.

saltatory

258. The chemical transmitter released at the motor end plate region is _____.

rheobase

259. The light bands seen in striated muscle are the _____ bands.

acetylcholine

260. The insulating material surrounding a nerve fiber is the _____ _____.

I

261. Muscle contraction without change in overall length is called _____ contraction.

myelin sheath

262. Increased frequency of nerve stimulation can result in a condition of the muscle called _____.

isometric

263. The contraction process involves the muscle proteins known as _____ and _____.

tetanus (tetany)

actin, myosin

You have completed Section II on Nerve-Muscle Physiology. Take a short break and then go on to Section III, which covers the physiology of the entire nervous system.

66

SECTION III

NERVOUS SYSTEM

The nervous system provides a means for the rapid transfer of information from one part of the body to another. Information about temperature, pressure, light, sound, position and other factors of our internal and external environment is transferred to the central nervous system for evaluation. Commands are issued by the central nervous system and carried to the body muscles for action.

The nervous system consists of the brain and spinal cord (comprising the central nervous system or CNS) and the peripheral nerves carrying information to and from the CNS. The function of the nervous system is closely related to its anatomy.

1. Nerves carrying information to the central

   _____ system are called sensory or afferent nerves.

2. The sensory nerves enter the spinal cord through   nervous
   the dorsal (posterior) nerve roots. (See illustration
   in Frame 7 to answer the next few frames.)

   The sensory nerve *cell bodies* lie outside of the

   spinal _____ in the dorsal root ganglia.

3. Nerves carrying information *from* the central   cord

   _____ _____ are termed motor or
   efferent nerves.

4. What kind of nerves carry information *to* the CNS?

5. The efferent, or _____, nerves leave the spinal cord via the ventral (anterior) nerve roots.

6. The motor nerve cell bodies lie within the

_____ cord.

7. A cross section of the spinal cord and its lateral connections on one side are shown in the following figure:

Spinal cord (posterior)
Dorsal
⊙ Nerve cell body
Dorsal root
Sensory neuron (afferent)
White matter
Gray matter
} Spinal nerve
Nerve cell
Ventral root
Motor neuron (efferent)
(Anterior)
Ventral

8. The spinal cord may be divided into *white matter*

(primarily nerve *fibers*) and _____ _____ (largely nerve *cell bodies*).

9. Sensory receptors in the skin, viscera, joints, muscles, and the special sense organs initiate sensory impulses. Different *sensory receptors* in the skin are sensitive to touch (tactile sensation), pain, and temperature. There is a special nervous pathway leading to the central nervous system for each

sensory _____.

10. The higher centers of the CNS interpret where the

stimulated sensory _____ are located on the body.

nervous system

afferent (sensory)

motor

spinal

gray matter

receptor

11. *Localization* is the term used to describe the association of a sensation with a particular part of the

_____ .

receptors

12. The term that indicates the association of a sensa-

tion with a part of the body is _____ .

body

13. When a stimulus is applied to a sensory _____
over a period of time, the sensation gradually
diminishes; this phenomenon is called *adaptation.*

localization

14. *Adaptation* implies two things. First, that a stimu-

lus is being applied over a period of _____ , and
that the sensation of this stimulus gradually

_____ .

receptor

15. Thus, when a stimulus is applied to a sensory receptor for a length of time and sensation dimin-

ishes, we can say that _____ has
occurred.

time
diminishes

16. A pain receptor in the viscera is a type of

_____ receptor.

adaptation

17. A proprioceptor is another type of sensory receptor that provides information about the degree of
muscle contraction or the position of a joint. Information about the position of a joint with
respect to the rest of the body is provided by

_____ .

sensory

18. Proprioceptor impulses enter the spinal column via
the (ventral/dorsal) root of the spinal nerve.

proprioceptors

69

19. After entering the spinal column, the proprioceptor impulses then ascend the _____ cord via neurons in a dorsal column and terminate in the *medulla.* Thus the proprioceptor impulses travel up the spinal cord through a _____ column and terminate in the _____.

dorsal
(impulses enter posteriorly)
(impulses leave anteriorly)

20. Let's review the pathway of proprioceptor impulses from their beginning. First, proprioceptors receive two kinds of information, one has to do with the degree of muscle _____, the other is concerned with the _____ of a joint. The proprioceptor impulses travel over the spinal nerve and enter the spinal column through the _____ root. Then the impulses ascend the spinal cord via _____ in the dorsal column and terminate in the _____.

spinal
dorsal
medulla

21. Now let's see what happens to these sensory impulses after they are received in the medulla. Other neurons connect with the sensory neuron terminations in the _____ and carry the impulses to the *thalamus* and the *sensory cortex* of the brain (on the opposite side of the body from which the impulse arose).

contraction
position
dorsal
neurons
medulla

22. Thus, after sensory impulses reach the medulla, they are conducted to two areas on the opposite side of the brain. These are the thalamus and _____ cortex.

medulla

23. Sensory fibers from pain and temperature receptors also enter the spinal cord via the dorsal _____ of the _____ nerve.

sensory

70

24. However, a second neuron in the spinal cord then picks up the signal, crosses to the opposite side of the _____ cord, and passes up a lateral column to the thalamus on that side.

root
spinal

25. In general, the sensory information received from one side of the body is transferred to the sensory cortex on the _____ side of the brain.

spinal

26. The proprioceptor neurons, which evaluate muscle _____, enter the dorsal root but *do not* cross to the other side in the spinal cord.

opposite

27. Proprioceptor neurons connect with other _____, which relay the information to the *cerebellum* for the coordination of muscular movement.

contraction

28. A part of the brain that coordinates muscular movement is the _____.

neurons

29. Collateral neurons connect the sensory tracts to the *reticular formation* of the brain where integration of sensory impulses occurs.

cerebellum

30. Destruction of the reticular formation in the brain leads to insensibility to _____ stimuli and to a deep sleep.

31. A part of the brain that *integrates* incoming sensory information is the _____ _____.

sensory

32. Certain anesthetics probably act by depressing the activity of the _____ formation.

reticular
formation

71

33. Now let's look at another part of the nervous system. The neurons carrying information to muscles for voluntary movement originate in the motor

    cortex of the _____.

reticular

34. Thus, neuronal impulses for voluntary muscle

    movement originate in the _____ _____.

brain

35. After the impulses are initiated, they travel down the *pyramidal tracts,* which connect the upper portions of the brain with the spinal cord, crossing over to the opposite side of the spinal cord and passing down the spinal cord to the cell bodies of motor neurons on that side. Thus, the right side of the body is controlled by the motor cortex on the (right/left) side of the brain. Likewise, the left side of the body is controlled by the right motor

    _____.

    Which motor cortex would you expect to be dominant in left-handed people?

motor cortex

36. The cells of motor neurons comprise the gray mat-

    ter of the _____ cord.

left
cortex
the right

37. Through branching of its axon, more than one hundred muscle fibers may be served by only one

    motor _____.

spinal

38. Each motor neuron has a cell body located in the gray matter called an *anterior horn cell.* An an-

    terior horn _____, its axon, and the muscle fibers it serves is called a motor unit.

neuron

39. As you learned earlier, the strength of a muscle contraction depends on the number of muscle fibers stimulated.

cell

40. The number of muscle _____ stimulated to contract depends on the number of anterior horn

cells that are _____.

41. Each _____ horn cell is acted on by many *neurons* in the spinal cord.

fibers
stimulated

42. Some of these _____ can stimulate an anterior horn cell.

anterior

43. Other neurons can inhibit the same _____

neurons

_____ _____.

44. Whether or not an anterior horn cell fires and initiates the contraction of its motor unit muscle fibers depends on the algebraic sum of the *stimulatory* and *inhibitory* effects of the other neurons on that cell. The stimulatory (+) and inhibitory (−) effects of neurons on an anterior horn cell in the

anterior
horn cell

spinal _____ are illustrated diagrammatically below:

DORSAL

White matter
Gray matter
Neurons from other parts of spinal cord
Anterior horn cell
Motor neuron

ANTERIOR

45. The neurons that act on an anterior horn cell may

cord

be motor _____ from higher centers or branches of sensory neurons.

46. Sensory neurons that enter the dorsal root of the

neurons

_____ _____ give off *branches* which

synapse with the anterior horn cells of the

_____ matter.

47. In the spinal cord *sensory* nerves enter the dorsal
root and give off *branches* that _____ with
the _____ _____ _____ .

spinal cord
gray

48. This relation between the _____ neurons
and the anterior horn _____ provides the
basis for the *spinal reflex.*

synapse
anterior horn cells

49. Spinal reflex pathways occur at the level of the

_____ _____ .

sensory
cells

50. For this reason, a decapitated animal can tempo-

rarily exhibit spinal _____ .

spinal cord

51. All along the spine, *sensory neurons* (enter/leave)
the spinal cord and *motor neurons* (enter/leave)
the spinal cord.

reflexes

52. A sensory impulse can give rise to a muscular contraction (reflex response) even if the spinal cord is
cut above the level at which the appropriate

_____ and _____ neurons enter and
leave. A spinal reflex pathway is shown below:

enter
leave

DORSAL

Sensory neuron from receptor

Synapse

Synapse

Anterior horn cell

Motor neuron to muscle

ANTERIOR

53. An example of a spinal *reflex* is the stretch *reflex.*
Muscles contain receptors, which are stimulated by
stretching. Thus these muscle receptors are called

_____ receptors.

sensory, motor

74

54. When the stretch _____ are stimulated   stretch
    they send sensory impulses over the dorsal root
    and into the spinal cord.

55. Within the spinal cord the sensory neuron from the   receptors
    stretch receptor synapses with one or more anterior

    _____ _____.

56. When the anterior horn cell is stimulated by *sen-*   horn cells

    sory impulses, it sends _____ impulses back
    to the muscle.

57. One stretch reflex, the knee-jerk _____, is   motor
    brought about by striking the patellar tendon.

58. The patellar tendon is attached to the quadriceps   reflex
    muscle, which extends the foreleg. Striking the
    patellar tendon causes the quadriceps muscle to

    stretch slightly, thus stimulating the _____

    _____ in the muscle.

59. The stretch receptors initiate a spinal _____,   stretch
    which results in kicking of the lower leg.   receptors

60. Spinal reflexes may be either excitatory or   reflex

    _____.

61. A reflex occurring on one side of the body may, by   inhibitory
    a connection in the spinal cord, inhibit or excite
    motor neurons on the other side of the body.

62. Thus, even if the spinal cord is cut between the
    brain and the level of a particular reflex pathway,
    stimulation of a sensory receptor in one leg (can/
    cannot) cause a reaction in the other leg.

63. An example of excitation and inhibition is the
crossed-extensor reflex illustrated in the following
figure:

can

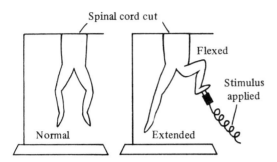

In this illustration a frog with only the lower spinal

_____ pathways present is given a stimulus
to one foot.

64. On the same side as the stimulus the motor nerves
of the extensor muscles are inhibited, thus the leg's
extensor muscles will (contract/relax). At the
same time the motor nerves to the flexor muscles
are excited, and therefore the flexor muscles will
(contract/relax).

reflex

65. However, in the opposite leg the extensor muscles

will _____ whereas the flexor muscles will

_____.

relax
contract

66. The overall action is a withdrawal of the stimulated

leg and _____ of the other leg.

contract
relax

67. The time taken for a reflex to occur depends on

how fast the neurons transmit the _____.

extension

68. Also included in the reflex time is the time it takes
for the impulse to jump from one neuron to another in the reflex pathway; that is, how long it

takes for the impulse to cross a _____.

impulses

69. Impulse conduction along a single _____ is very fast.

synapse

70. But, an impulse is slowed down at the junction of two neurons or, in other words, at the _____.

neuron

71. In summary, synaptic transmission is (slower/faster) than nerve conduction and is thus the rate-limiting step in a reflex pathway.

synapse

72. A spinal reflex can occur even if the animal's brain has been _____.

slower

73. However, under normal conditions the brain does influence _____ reflexes, either reinforcing or inhibiting them.

removed (severed, destroyed, mushed, etc.)

74. The usual influence by the _____ is to inhibit (but not eliminate) spinal reflexes.

spinal

75. The stretch receptors of muscles are activated by a change in the _____ of the muscle.

brain (higher centers)

76. In addition, these _____ receptors are acted upon by special muscles attached directly in series with the receptors.

length

77. These special *muscles* are called intrafusal _____.

stretch

78. The intrafusal muscles together with a stretch _____ is termed the *muscle spindle.*

muscles

79. The stretch receptor together with the attached intrafusal muscles form the _____ _____.

receptor

80. A special neuronal pathway to the muscle called the γ (gamma) *motor neuron* stimulates the intrafusal _____ to contract.

muscle spindle

81. The intrafusal muscles contract after stimulation
by the _____ motor neuron.

muscles

82. A *muscle spindle* and its neuronal connections are shown in the next illustration.

gamma (γ)

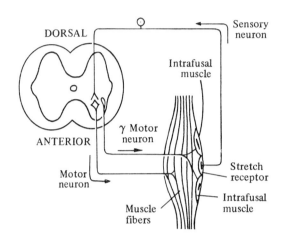

The intrafusal muscles together with a stretch receptor comprise a muscle _____.

83. Upon stimulation the gamma motor neurons cause contraction of the _____ muscle fibers.

spindle

84. Contraction of the _____ _____ fibers stimulates the attached stretch receptors.

intrafusal

85. The stretch receptors initiate the stretch _____ just discussed, causing contraction of the main muscle fibers.

intrafusal muscle

86. This in turn reduces the tension on the muscle spindle and on the stretch _____.

reflex

87. The muscle spindles and gamma motor neurons provide a means of fine control for muscle action.

   The fine reflex control offered by the _____

   spindles and the _____ motor neurons is evident in the ability to maintain a limb at a precise point in space.

   receptor

88. One of the major problems posed to the nervous system is maintaining balance while moving the body. Information about body position, balance, and motion is conveyed to the CNS from *proprioceptors* in the muscles and joints. Proprioceptors of the upper cervical region provide information about head position which is used to prepare the body muscles for an expected movement or for regaining an upright position. On either side of the head deeply embedded in the walls of the skull are two important proprioceptors, called the *labyrinths*.

   These special proprioceptors on either side of the head are called the _____ .

   muscle
   gamma (γ)

89. The labyrinths are closely related anatomically to the cochlea, that part of the inner ear which acts as a receptor for sound. These proprioceptors, called

   _____ consist of three semicircular canals lying in three planes of space approximately at right angles to one another.

   labyrinths

90. In addition to the membrane-lined semicircular _____ , the labyrinths also have two membranous sacs, the *utricle* and the *saccule*.

   labyrinths

91. The labyrinth consists of three semicircular canals and two membranous sacs, the utricle and the

   _____ .

   canals

79

92. The utricle is continuous with the ends of each

_____ canal.

saccule

93. Both the utricle and the _____ contain
sensory receptors consisting of an epithelium containing hair cells.

semicircular

94. Both the utricle and the saccule contain _____
receptors.

saccule

95. The hair cells of the _____ and saccule
epithelia are overlaid by a gelatinous mass in which
many small calcareous nodules, called the *otoliths*
or *ear stones* are embedded.

sensory

96. Above the hair cells of the _____ and

_____ are the ear stones or otoliths.

utricle

97. When the head moves, the ear stones or _____
and gelatinous mass move the hairs (cilia) of the
epithelial cells.

utricle
saccule

98. Sensory nerves surround the bases of the hair cells
and are stimulated by the movement of the hairs.
This principle is illustrated in the diagram below:

otoliths

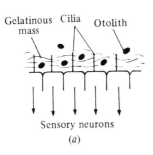

(a)

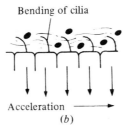

(b)

As the body attains a constant *velocity* the cilia
(hairs) return to their normal position and the sen-

sory _____ from the cells decrease.

99. The utricle and saccule, then, are sensitive to changes in velocity—that is, *acceleration.*

impulses

100. The semicircular _____ are fluid-filled.

101. Each canal contains a sensory area that can detect the movement of the _____ within the canal.

canals

102. When the body is rotated, the fluid in a canal moves relative to the canal wall. The canal most affected will be the one located in the plane of the body's _____.

fluid

103. This principle is shown in the next diagram:

rotation

Fluid   Receptor   Receptor bent   Sensory neuron

Sensory neuron   Relative movement of fluid

(a) At rest   (b) Rotation of wall

When the body rotates quickly, the canal fluid moves more slowly than the canal wall due to inertia of the fluid. This bends the sensory receptors in a direction opposite to that of body rotation.

104. The relative movement of fluid in the canal activates the sensory _____ of that canal.

105. The stimulated sensory receptors provide the CNS with information about the direction of _____ which caused the fluid movement.

receptors (neurons)

106. Rotation of the body in one plane activates the sensory receptors of the semicircular canal located in that _____.

rotation

81

107. Now let's discuss how the eye provides visual information about the position and motion of the body. The eye is basically a *lens* system with a light recording area. Light, which normally travels in a

straight line, is bent or refracted by a _____.

plane

108. Light refraction is illustrated for two types of lenses in the next figure:

lens

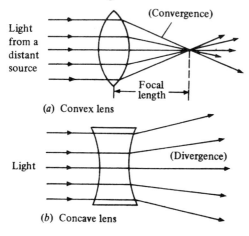

(Convergence)

Light from a distant source

Focal length

(*a*) Convex lens

(Divergence)

Light

(*b*) Concave lens

Refer to this illustration to complete the next few frames. The distance from the center of the lens to the point at which the light rays converge is

called the _____ _____.

109. The thicker a convex lens is, the shorter will be its _____ length.

focal length

110. The image produced by a convex _____ is inverted as shown in the next diagram.

focal

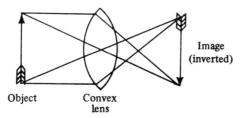

Image (inverted)

Object   Convex lens

82

111. The *power* of a lens is expressed in *diopters* and is equal to the reciprocal of the _____ length (expressed in meters).

lens

112. In other words

$$\frac{?}{} = \frac{1}{\text{focal length}}$$

focal

113. What is the *power* in *diopters* of a lens whose focal length is 0.5 meters?

power (of a lens)

114. The eye contains two lenses, the lens proper and the cornea. The combined power of these lenses is about +59 _____.

2 diopters

115. Since the lens system of the eye acts as a convex lens, the image it focuses on the *retina* is _____.

diopters

116. The eye focuses an image by changing the curvature (convexity) of the _____ and thereby changing its power.

inverted

117. *Accommodation* is the term used to describe the action that changes the power of the _____.

lens

118. The ability of the eye to become more convex and thus increase its power decreases with age. With age there is a loss of _____.

lens

119. The *ciliary muscles* of the eye bring about accommodation. The muscles responsible for accommodation of the eye are the _____ muscles.

accommodation

120. The lens of a young person is elastic and tends to assume a more spherical _____. A lens that is more spherical is *thicker* through the center than a flattened lens. Therefore, which lens is more powerful?

ciliary

121. Ligaments attached to the edge of the lens prevent it from attaining a _____ shape.

shape
the more spherical (convex) lens

122. Contraction of the ciliary muscles releases the tension on the ligaments attached to the lens, thereby allowing the lens to assume a more _____ shape.

spherical

123. Does contraction of the ciliary muscles increase or decrease the power of the lens?

spherical

124. *Presbyopia* is a term for the inability of the lens to increase its power. That is, the eye is unable to _____ even though the _____ muscles relax the ligaments.

increases

125. Accommodation is a reflex brought about through the central _____ system.

accommodate, ciliary

126. The term *depth of focus* describes the ability of the eye to focus on objects at different distances from the eye at the same time. The ability of the eye to focus simultaneously on objects at different distances from the eye is called the eye's _____ of _____.

nervous

127. The size of the pupillary aperture (i.e., the iris) determines both the amount of light that enters the eye and the _____ of _____.

depth
focus

128. The central nervous system controls the size of the pupillary aperture or the _____ by reflex.

depth, focus

129. Imperfections of the lens system distort the image cast on the light sensitive surface of the eye, called the retina. Several of these refractive errors are illustrated on the following page.

iris

84

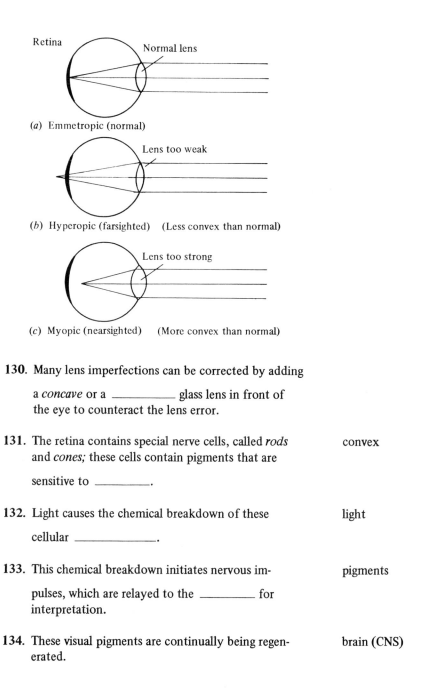

(a) Emmetropic (normal)

(b) Hyperopic (farsighted)   (Less convex than normal)

(c) Myopic (nearsighted)   (More convex than normal)

130. Many lens imperfections can be corrected by adding a *concave* or a _____ glass lens in front of the eye to counteract the lens error.

131. The retina contains special nerve cells, called *rods* and *cones;* these cells contain pigments that are sensitive to _____.

convex

132. Light causes the chemical breakdown of these cellular _____.

light

133. This chemical breakdown initiates nervous impulses, which are relayed to the _____ for interpretation.

pigments

134. These visual pigments are continually being regenerated.

brain (CNS)

135. We are now going to discuss the next function of the nervous system–hearing. Hearing is brought about by sound waves causing the ear drum or tympanic membrane to vibrate. This vibration is transferred through a system of bony levers (malleus, incus, and stapes, together called the ossicles) in the middle ear to the *cochlea,* which contains receptors sensitive to vibration. The amount of sound reaching the inner chamber, the cochlea, can be regulated by muscles attached to the ossicles of

the middle _____.

136. The inner chamber or _____ is filled with fluid and is divided by a partition called the *basilar membrane.*

ear

137. The cochlea is filled with fluid and is divided by

the _____ _____.

cochlea

138. The basilar _____ contains *hair cells* with closely associated *sensory receptors.*

basilar membrane

139. These sensory receptors are sensitive to vibration

of the _____, which fills the cochlea.

membrane

140. Sound vibration is transferred by the ossicles (middle ear) to the cochlea (_____ ear).

fluid

141. This transfer of vibration occurs as the ossicles of the middle ear vibrate against a small membrane covering an opening to the fluid-filled inner ear, or

the _____.

inner

142. Depending on the frequency of the sound, certain

hair cells on the basilar _____ located within the cochlea resonate.

cochlea

143. The resonating _____ cells send impulses to the CNS.

membrane

144. The pitch (frequency) of a sound is interpreted according to which _____ cells are stimulated.

    hair

145. The loudness of a sound is related to the *number* of _____ _____ in a particular group that are stimulated.

    hair

146. The particular hair cells that are stimulated will determine the _____ of a sound. And the loudness of a sound depends on the _____ of hair cells stimulated in a particular group.

    hair cells

147. The frequency of a sound is related to the rate of *vibration* (cycles per second, or cps) of the sound. Loudness depends on the energy of the sound vibration, which is measured in decibels.

The energy of a sound is measured in _____.

    frequency (pitch)
    number

148. Loudness depends on the _____ of the sound vibration, which is measured in _____.

    decibels

149. Whether or not a sound can be heard depends on both its frequency and its loudness, as shown in the next graph:

    energy
    decibels

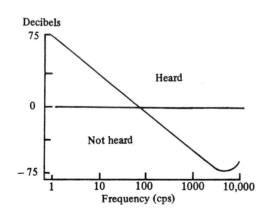

Can a zero decibel sound be heard if its frequency is 1000 cps? If its frequency is 10 cps?

150. The normal audible *frequency* range at zero decibels is about 30 to 20,000 _____.

yes, no

151. We've discussed several functions of the CNS; now let's discuss various functions of an important part of the peripheral nervous system, the autonomic nervous system. A part of the peripheral nervous system that acts on the viscera, on the *glands* of secretion, and on involuntary (smooth) *muscle* is called the *autonomic* nervous system. The sympathetic system and the parasympathetic system are

the divisions of the _____ nervous system.

cps

152. Both of these subdivisions of the _____ nervous system are efferent (i.e., motor) systems.

autonomic

153. *Sensory* nerves carry impulses (to/from) the CNS; *motor* nerves carry impulses (to/from) the CNS.

autonomic

154. Autonomic nerves are all efferent. That is, they carry information (to/from) muscles, glands, and viscera.

to
from

155. Autonomic nerves are classed as either sympathetic

or _____.

to

156. The sympathetic nerve fibers leave the CNS in the

thoracic and upper lumbar regions of the _____ cord.

parasympathetic

157. The other autonomic nerves, the _____ nerves, leave the CNS via cranial nerves (III, V, VII, IX, and X) and at the sacral region of the spinal cord.

spinal

88

158. The sympathetic neurons arise in the _____ matter of the spinal cord and leave the cord via ventral roots.

parasympathetic

159. Once out of the spinal cord these neurons synapse with other _____, which carry impulses to an effector somewhere in the body.

gray

160. Parallel to the spinal column on each side are long *chains* of *synapses* of sympathetic nerves. These chains of _____ occur where nerve axons from cells inside the spinal cord join with nerve cells of other neurons outside the spinal cord. This arrangement for one side of the spinal cord is shown below:

neurons

Preganglionic neurons

Postganglionic neurons

Ganglion

Innervated organ

Spinal cord

Sympathetic chain

161. Refer to the illustration to complete the next few frames. The thick parts of the chains of _____ occur at each spinal segment and are called ganglia. One is called a _____.

synapses

162. The thick parts of the chains of synapses are called _____. The neurons leading from the spinal cord to the ganglia are called _____

synapses
ganglion.

89

163. The neurons leading from a ganglion to an innervated structure are called _____

_____.

164. The *para*sympathetic system also contains preganglionic and _____ neurons.

165. However, in the parasympathetic system most preganglionic fibers extend all the way to the innervated _____.

166. The pre- and postganglionic fibers still synapse, but
the synapse usually lies within the innervated structure. Thus, in the parasympathetic system the preganglionic fibers are usually (short/long) and the
postganglionic fibers are quite (short/long).

167. The activity of the autonomic system is normally
controlled by the brain, primarily the cerebral cortex, the hypothalamus, and the medulla. The chemical transmitter substance at the preganglionic–
postganglionic synapses of both sympathetic

and _____ systems is acetylcholine.

168. A ganglionic blocking agent can prevent the transmission of _____ across these synapses.

169. The chemical transmitter substance acting between
a parasympathetic postganglionic neuron and an
innervated organ is also acetylcholine. In most of
the sympathetic system the chemical transmitter
between the postganglionic neuron and the inner-

vated _____ is norepinephrine.

170. The neurons that release _____
are termed *adrenergic.*

171. The neurons that release norepinephrine are called

    _____.

172. The parasympathetic postganglionic neurons re-

    lease _____.

173. These acetylcholine-releasing neurons are termed

    cholinergic _____.

174. Neurons that release acetylcholine are

    _____ neurons.

175. In general the sympathetic nervous system is acti-
    vated by stressful situations requiring sudden and
    vigorous action. Therefore, which autonomic
    nerves are responsible for fight-or-flight responses?

176. Which nerves prepare the body for sudden and
    vigorous action?

177. The other division of the autonomic system is
    more diversified in its activities, controlling many
    different bodily functions. This is the

    _____ system.

178. Most organs of the body are innervated by both

    the _____ and _____
    divisions of the autonomic system although the
    supply to a particular organ may be predominantly
    one or the other.

179. The actions induced in a structure by each auto-
    nomic division are usually opposite. Some of these
    actions are listed in the following table (dashed
    lines indicate little or no effect).

norepinephrine

adrenergic

acetylcholine

neurons

cholinergic

sympathetic

sympathetic

parasympathetic

sympathetic
parasympathetic

91

ORGAN	SYMPATHETIC EFFECT	PARASYMPATHETIC EFFECT
heart	increases heart rate	decreases heart rate
gastrointes- tinal tract	inhibits food movement	increases food movement
blood vessels	vasoconstriction (in skin) vasoconstriction (in muscles)	————————
pancreas	————————	increased secretion
sweat glands	increased sweat production	————————
eye	dilates pupil	constricts pupil
bronchi	dilates	constricts
bladder	————————	empties

180. In the remaining frames of this section we'll discuss the anatomical and functional relationships of
a few important brain structures.

The brain is divided into several major portions;
the medulla, pons, thalamus, hypothalamus, cerebellum, and cerebrum. Locate these structures in
the following diagram.

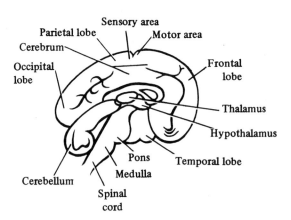

181. Refer to the illustration and complete the next few frames.

The *cerebrum* is subdivided into the frontal, parietal, occipital, and temporal _____.

182. Sensory impulses travel up the spinal cord to centers in the medulla and, immediately above, in the

_____.

lobes

183. The centers in the _____ and _____ reflexly respond to sensory impulses by initiating appropriate motor responses.

pons

184. Centers that regulate heart rate, respiratory muscles, swallowing, and the sizes of blood vessels (vasomotor reflexes) are located in the central area of the pons and medulla, and are called the *reticular formation*.

medulla, pons

185. The inner core of the medulla and pons is called the _____ _____.

186. The centers in the reticular formation are sensitive to changes in blood carbon dioxide, blood pH, and to various drugs carried to the areas by the circulation. The activity of the reticular breathing centers varies with blood carbon dioxide; the vomiting center responds to various emetics such as apomorphine and ipecac by initiating the vomiting reflex.

reticular formation

187. The reticular formation, when stimulated, produces an "arousal" reaction in the individual, alerting the individual and maintaining his attention. It is also concerned with specific control of muscular activity and with the maintenance of tone in the postural muscles. This area probably constitutes the most important regulatory mechanism of the central nervous system.

188. The *thalamus* is the major site for sorting and interpreting sensory impulses from the widespread receptors of the body. Sorted impulses are relayed

from the _____ to the cerebrum.

189. One function of the *hypothalamus* is the reflex regulation of body temperature. Through its effect on blood vessel dilation in the skin, water loss, and metabolism, the hypothalamus regulates body

_____.

thalamus

190. Another function of the _____ is the *integration* of sympathetic and parasympathetic nervous activity.

temperature

191. Thus, we say that the hypothalamus integrates

_____ and _____ nervous activity.

hypothalamus

192. The hypothalamus exerts additional regulatory effects through its action on the pituitary

_____ (to be covered in the endocrine section).

sympathetic
parasympathetic

193. Look again at the illustration in Frame 180. Beneath the occipital lobe of the cerebrum lies the

_____.

gland

194. The modulation (augmentation or inhibition) of muscular movements is the chief role of the

_____.

cerebellum

195. Thus, jerky muscular activity and an inability to bring about fine coordinated movements can result from

damage to the _____.

cerebellum

196. Rapid growth during development at the surface of the brain (the cortical part of the _____) produces foldings or convolutions.

cerebellum

197. The cerebral cortex contains *sensory* and *motor* areas. The sensations of heat, light, cold, etc., can be elicited by electrical stimulation of the

_____ areas of the cerebral cortex.

cerebrum

198. Which cerebral cortex areas could be experimentally stimulated to induce various motor responses?

sensory

199. Information gained from the experimental stimulation of various parts of the _____ cortex has been used to "map" the cortex.

motor areas

200. "Mapping" involves the localization of areas of the

_____ _____ related to specific functions.

cerebral

201. You will notice in the illustration in Frame 180 that the *motor* areas of the cortex are located in the frontal lobe at the central fold separating the

frontal and _____ lobes.

cerebral cortex

202. Stimulation of this _____ area produces well-integrated movements of a given limb, that is, not just a single muscle movement.

parietal

203. Just behind the motor area, in the parietal lobe, is

the _____ area.

motor

204. Part of the *temporal* lobe is concerned with hearing, receiving sensory impulses from the inner ear

chamber called the _____.

sensory

205. Impulses from the cochlea are received in the

_____ lobe.

cochlea

206. The *occipital lobe* of the *cerebrum* interprets visual stimuli. The part of the cerebrum where visual

stimuli are interpreted is the _____ _____.

temporal

207. The inner bulk of the cerebrum consists of associa-   occipital lobe
tion areas related to the interpretation of sensory
impulses (learning, reasoning, etc.).

You have completed Section III, covering the physiology of the nervous system.
In the next section we'll discuss the functions and relationships within the cardiovascular system.

CARDIOVASCULAR SYSTEM

The circulation of blood in the body occurs essentially by means of two pumps (the left and right sides of the heart) and two sets of tubes (the systemic circulation and the pulmonary circulation) all connected in series. Both the systemic and the pulmonary circuits are subdivided into many parallel circuits such as branches serving the kidneys, the intestines, each leg, etc.

Circulating blood carries oxygen from the lungs to the tissues and carbon dioxide from the tissues to the lungs. It also transports food from the digestive tract to the tissues and waste products from the tissues to the kidneys for excretion. In addition, circulating blood distributes drugs and hormones to the tissues on which they act.

1. A 70-kilogram adult man has a blood volume of about 5 liters. At any given time about one-fifth of this blood (what volume?) will be in his lung capillaries, 3 liters in his systemic veins, and 1 liter in his heart and systemic arteries and capillaries.

2. If blood is prevented from clotting, perhaps with heparin, and allowed to stand in a test tube, the cellular constituents will settle to the bottom under the influence of gravity. This process is speeded up by centrifugation. The diagram on the following page shows the layers obtained by spinning blood in a centrifuge. Refer to this illustration for the next few frames.

1 liter

97

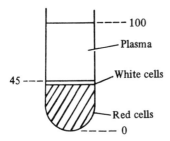

Which are more dense, red cells (erythrocytes) or white cells?

3. About what per cent of total blood volume do the cellular constituents of this blood sample occupy?

    red cells

4. Almost all of this cellular volume consists of

    _____ cells.

    about 45%

5. The small intermediate layer known as the buffy coat is formed by the less dense _____ cells.

    red

6. The top layer of the sample consists of a straw colored fluid called _____.

    white

7. The per cent of the total volume occupied by red _____ is called the *hematocrit* or packed cell volume. The normal range is 40 to 47%.

    plasma

8. In every cubic millimeter (mm^3) of blood there are about 5 million red _____ _____ (RBC's).

    cells

9. Red _____ contain the pigment hemoglobin (Hb), which enables them to carry oxygen.

    blood cells

10. The pigment that enables red blood cells to carry oxygen is _____.

    cells

11. Red cells also contain the enzyme *carbonic anhy-drase,* which is important in the transport of carbon dioxide. The enzyme in red cells related to carbon dioxide (CO_2) transport is _____ _____.

hemoglobin (Hb)

12. Hemoglobin contains iron in the ferrous form. The iron of hemoglobin combines loosely with oxygen: the iron *remains* in the _____ form. This process is called oxygenation.

carbonic anhydrase

13. If the hemoglobin molecule becomes *oxidized* (i.e., the iron is converted from the *ferrous* state to the *ferric* state), hemoglobin is no longer effective in _____ transport.

ferrous

14. Oxidized hemoglobin is called *methemoglobin* and contains _____ in the ferric state.

oxygen

15. One gram of hemoglobin combines loosely with 1.34 ml of oxygen. A normal adult has about 14.5 grams of hemoglobin per 100 ml of blood. Compute the volume of oxygen which each 100 ml of blood can carry:

iron

16. Reduced hemoglobin has a dark red color because it is not combined with _____.

(14.5g Hb/100 ml blood) X (1.34 ml O_2/g Hb) = 19.4 ml O_2

17. Hemoglobin loosely combined with oxygen is called oxyhemoglobin and its color is light _____.

oxygen (O_2)

18. What color is blood when it arrives at the lungs?

red

19. In passing through the lungs, 95 to 100% of the blood's hemoglobin combines with _____, making the blood turn light _____.

dark red

99

20. The blood then returns to the tissue capillaries where _____ leaves the blood and _____ _____ enters the blood.

O_2
red

21. Venous blood contains less oxygen and is (what color?) _____ _____. Then it returns to the _____ for more _____.

oxygen, carbon dioxide

22. If the blood does not absorb enough oxygen on its passage through the lungs then the arterial blood will also be _____ _____.

dark red
lungs, oxygen

23. An individual becomes visibly blue and is said to be *cyanosed* if less than 95% of the arterial hemoglobin is combined with _____ after its passage through the lungs.

dark red

24. Cyanosis results from a (high/low) oxygen saturation of the hemoglobin. The _____ red blood appears blue through the blood vessel walls.

oxygen

25. A red cell has a life span of about 120 days after which time it breaks down and is replaced by a new cell. About how many months does a red cell live?

low
dark

26. Red cells, or erythrocytes, are formed from reticulo-endothelial cells within bone marrow. The genesis of a red cell (erythropoiesis) involves the following steps: proerythroblast → normoblast → reticulocyte → red cell, which is also called an

_____.

4

27. The developing red cells have nuclei but the final red cells have no _____.

erythrocyte

28. A deficiency of red cell production is a type of *aplastic anemia.* Thus, when blood tests indicate that an individual's red cell production has decreased, he is said to suffer from a condition called

_____ _____.

nuclei

29. The formation of new red blood cells requires an adequate diet. What mineral element have we already mentioned as important to red cell oxygen transport?

aplastic anemia

30. Much of the iron from broken down erythrocytes

is reused in the formation of new _____.

iron

31. The daily dietary requirement for a man is about 5 mg of iron. Because the menstrual flow represents an absolute loss of iron, women require about

twice this much iron per day or about _____mg per day.

erythrocytes (red blood cells)

32. A dietary iron deficiency will lead to red cells that are (poor/rich) in iron?

10 mg

33. Iron deficiency results in *hypochromic anemia.* Which are more likely to be affected, men or women?

poor

34. Two additional substances are necessary for the normal formation of red blood cells. These are vitamin B_{12} and an *"intrinsic factor"* produced by the stomach. Thus, the hematopoetic factor is a combination of the intrinsic factor and vitamin

_____.

women

35. Vitamin B_{12}, when present in the diet, is absorbed from the intestine. The intrinsic factor facilitates

the absorption of vitamin B_{12} from the _____.

B_{12}

101

36. Thus, a vitamin B_{12} deficiency may occur for either of two reasons. B_{12} may be absent from the diet or the intestine may be unable to absorb it due to

    a lack of the _____ factor.

    intestine

37. Lack of vitamin B_{12} results in red cells that are deficient both in number and in quality. This condition should be recognized as another type of

    _____.

    intrinsic

38. If untreated, this anemic condition is often fatal

    and is thus termed pernicious _____.

    anemia

39. The stimulus for increased erythrocyte formation is a low oxygen pressure. This is more likely to occur at (higher/lower) altitudes.

    anemia

40. The reticulo-endothelial system removes broken down red cells from the circulation. The iron re-

    moved from broken down _____ _____ is stored for future use as *ferritin*.

    higher

41. The protein of the red cell is broken down to *amino acids*, which may be utilized to build more proteins in the body.

    red cells

42. Finally, the pigment portion of the hemoglobin molecule is converted to the yellow *pigment bilirubin* and the green _____ *biliverdin*. (These colors often appear through the skin as the dark reduced hemoglobin is converted to the yel-

    low pigment _____, and the green pig-

    ment _____ in a bruise.)

43. These pigments pass from the blood to the *liver*.

    From the _____ they are transferred to the bile duct and into the duodenum. They are excreted in the feces.

    pigment
bilirubin
biliverdin

102

44. Any blockage of the bilirubin excretory pathway will result in an accumulation of bilirubin in the

_____.

liver

45. Bilirubin is a yellow _____. When its concentration in the blood becomes very high, the patient's skin and eyes assume a _____ color—a condition called *jaundice*.

blood

46. Blood plasma is about 91% water. *Plasma* proteins constitute about 7% of plasma. Also present are inorganic salts, such as sodium chloride and bicarbonate, plus such materials being transported in the blood as glucose. The plasma proteins are albumin, globulin, prothrombin, and fibrinogen. The viscosity of *plasma* depends on the size and shape of

these _____ in the plasma.

pigment
yellow

47. The plasma proteins can combine with both acids and alkalis and therefore can prevent large changes

in the acidity of the _____.

proteins

48. Substances that inhibit changes in acidity are called *buffers*. Since the plasma *proteins* inhibit changes

in acidity, they may be called _____.

plasma (blood)

49. In addition to red cells (erythrocytes) the blood

also contains white _____ (called leucocytes) and platelets.

buffers

50. There are several different types of leucocytes (WBC's). For example:

Lymphocytes   Granulocytes
Monocytes   (of which there are three type)
                 neutrophils   basophils
                 eosinophils

cells

White blood cells (WBC's) or _____
are important in the control of infections through their "phagocytic" action.

51. Phagocytes are cells that may engulf and destroy foreign matter or harmful bacteria.

Certain types of leucocytes that can engulf foreign

matter or bacteria are called _____.

Platelets are essential to the clotting of _____.

leucocytes

52. Blood clots when the soluble plasma protein, *fibrinogen,* changes into the insoluble *fibrin.* Thus

blood clots when _____ changes into

_____.

phagocytes
blood

53. Fibrin forms a network of thin strands that entrap the solid elements of blood, chiefly RBC's. The

entrapment of these elements forms a _____.

fibrinogen
fibrin

54. The soft *clot* that is formed gradually contracts or shrinks and exudes a fluid called *serum.*

When the soft clot contracts, it exudes _____.

clot

55. Another protein, thrombin, causes fibrinogen to

change into _____.

serum

56. Fibrinogen changes into fibrin due to the influence

of _____.

fibrin

57. Thrombin in turn had to be produced from pro-thrombin in the presence of *thromboplastin* and calcium ions.

Thrombin is produced from prothrombin in the

presence of _____ ions and _____.

thrombin

58. Thromboplastin is formed when the blood platelets break down *and* when tissue is damaged.

When is thromboplastin formed?

calcium, thromboplastin

59. The major steps in blood clotting are:

Platelet breakdown or tissue damage

↓

Prothrombin + thromboplastin + Ca^{+2}

↓

Fibrinogen + thrombin → fibrin

when platelets break down or tissue is damaged

60. A clot occurring in the circulation is called a *thrombus.* Stroke is a condition that may result

when a clot or _____ occurs in the brain.

61. A thrombus that becomes detached from its site of formation and free to travel through the

_____ is called an *embolus.*

thrombus

62. A pulmonary embolism refers to an embolus that

has _____ to the lungs and become lodged in one of the pulmonary capillaries.

circulation (blood vessels)

63. The use of anticoagulants to prevent *clotting* depends on the interruption of one or more of the clotting steps. For example, since Ca^{+2} is necessary for clotting, drawn blood may be prevented

from _____ by adding a fluoride, oxalate,

or citrate to precipitate _____.

circulated (traveled)

64. Heparin prevents clotting by inhibiting the conver-

sion of prothrombin to _____.

clotting
Ca^{+2}

65. Substances such as dicoumarol and phenidione prevent clotting by (decreasing/increasing) the formation of prothrombin.

thrombin

66. Blood typing is based on a reaction between red cells and plasma. Many typing systems exist (Rh, MN, etc.). One of the most important systems with respect to blood transfusion is the ABO system described next.

decreasing

An agglutinogen is a cellular substance which may participate in a reaction causing a clumping together or *agglutination* of red cells.

Cellular substances participating in red _____ clumping, or _____, are called

_____.

67. Two types of these substances are termed *agglutinogens* A and B. They define a person's ABO blood type. Thus, a person whose red cells have only

    agglutinogen A has type ___ blood. And a person having red cells with only the B agglutinogen has

    type ___ blood.

    cell
    agglutination
    agglutinogens

68. What agglutinogens are found on the erythrocytes of people with type AB blood?

    A
    B

69. A person whose red cells have neither A nor B agglutinogens has blood type O.

    Plasma may contain substances which by reacting with the cell agglutinogens cause the red cells to

    clump together, or _____.

    both A and B
    agglutinogens

70. Clumped or _____ cells may block small capillaries and lead to the death of the tissues served by these capillaries.

    agglutinate

71. Plasma substances causing agglutination are called *agglutinins*. In the ABO system these are anti-A

    agglutinin and anti-B _____.

    agglutinated

72. Anti-A agglutinin causes clumping of red cells having agglutinogen A. Therefore, what blood types would show clumping on the addition of anti-B agglutinin?

    agglutinin

73. Anti-A agglutinin is found in the plasma of persons having type B or type O red cells. Therefore, anti-B

    is found in the plasma of persons having type ___

    or type ___ red cells.

    types B and AB

106

74. Below is a summary of the ABO types:

A

O

Type	O	A	B	AB
cell agglutinogen	—	A	B	A & B
plasma agglutinin	anti-A & anti-B	anti-B	anti-A	—

A transfusion of mismatched blood may result in severe kidney damage and death. This is due to the

clumping or _____ of the donated cells.

75. Now let's take a look at the system that circulates the blood. The general scheme of the circulatory system is illustrated below. Use this diagram to complete the next few frames.

agglutination

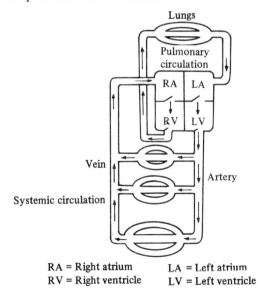

RA = Right atrium   LA = Left atrium
RV = Right ventricle   LV = Left ventricle

Blood flows from the left ventricle of the heart, through the systemic circulation, and returns to

the _____ atrium and then into the right

_____.

76. From the right ventricle blood flows to the

_____ and returns to the _____ _____

and from there into the _____ _____ .

right
ventricle

77. Blood flow, which is a function of pressure and of resistance, is an amount (volume) of blood moved per unit time.

Blood flow is a function of _____ and

_____ .

lungs, left atrium
left ventricle

78. _Pressure_ is a force applied to an area.

When the heart contracts it exerts _____ on the blood within it.

pressure
resistance

79. Pressure exerted by the heart forces _____ through the arterial branches.

pressure

80. The _total resistance_ offered the blood by the circulation is called the _peripheral resistance_ (PR). Changing the size of the body's arterioles changes

the magnitude of the PR (_____ resist-ance).

blood

81. Contraction of smooth muscle around the _arterioles_ makes these vessels (smaller/larger).

peripheral

82. The *vasomotor* center in the *medulla* controls the smooth muscle around each _____.

smaller

83. The smooth muscle around the arterioles is controlled by the _____ center in the _____.

arteriole

84. An *increase* in vasomotor activity decreases the radii of the _____. This is vasoconstriction.

vasomotor
medulla

85. The process of vasodilation is a *decrease* of vasomotor activity, which leads to a(n) (increase/decrease) in arteriolar size.

arterioles

86. Thus an increase in arteriole size is called _____. A decrease in arteriole size is called _____.

increase

87. The *flow* through a blood vessel is equal to the effective *blood pressure* (BP) divided by the *resistance* to flow. The basic relationship is summarized in the following formula:

$$\text{Flow} = \frac{\text{Arterial BP} - \text{Venous BP}}{\text{Peripheral resistance}}$$

At the heart, the blood *flow* equals the *arterial* blood _____ divided by the _____ *resistance.*

vasodilation
vasoconstriction

88. Both the systemic circulation and the *pulmonary* _____ occur through the following sequence of vessels: arteries, arterioles, capillaries, venules, and veins.

pressure, peripheral
(total)

89. The flow leaving the heart equals the flow returning to the _____.

circulation

109

90. However, the flow in an individual capillary is much (greater/smaller) than that in a large artery.

91. The resistance to flow in a vessel is *inversely* proportional to the cross-sectional area of that vessel. Thus, the smaller the cross-sectional area, the

   higher the _____ to flow.

92. Each *capillary* has a very small cross section: its resistance is (low/high) and consequently its flow is (small/great).

93. Nevertheless, the *total* cross-sectional area of all the capillaries is (large/small).

94. The total flow (the sum of the individual capillary flows) is equal to the flow leaving and returning to

   the _____.

95. The blood pressures shown in the figure below are average values for the systemic circulation for a normal person in the horizontal position. The illustration shows that the blood pressure decreases with a(n) (decrease/increase) in distance from the heart.

heart

smaller

resistance

high
small

large

heart

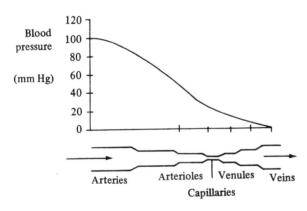

96. What effect on blood pressure has to be considered in the vertical position?

increase

110

97. The average pressure of the _____ leaving the *right side* of the _____ (i.e., in the pulmonary artery) is about 14 mm Hg.

gravity

98. In the vertical position the pressure of blood below the heart (abdomen, legs, feet, etc.) will be (increased/decreased) due to the weight of the blood above the point of measurement.

blood
heart

99. This increase in _____ is directly proportional to the distance below the heart.

increased

100. If the average blood pressure at the heart were 100 mm Hg, about 170 mm Hg would be the

_____ in the feet.

pressure

101. While standing, the pressures above the heart are (greater/less) than the pressure at the heart.

pressure

102. High gravitational forces such as those produced by acceleration can decrease the blood pressure in the brain sufficiently to cause a blackout or increase it enough to cause hemorrhage (red-out). The effect produced—blackout or red-out—would depend on the body's position relative to the gravitational forces.

less

103. The heart is composed of *cardiac muscle* which has an inherent rhythmicity. This property of rhythmic contraction is most highly developed in an area of the right atrium called the sino-atrial node (S-A node). Because it normally initiates the heartbeat, the pacemaker is another name for the

_____ - _____ node.

104. The area of the heart that normally begins each heartbeat is called the _____ - _____ node or the _____.

sino-atrial (S-A)

111

105. As we noted earlier, muscle excitation is accomplished through the *depolarization* of the muscle cell membrane. Excitation of the heart muscle

normally begins at the _____-_____ node and spreads to all parts of the heart as a wave of depolarization.

106. The path of the *depolarization* wave over the heart musculature is diagramed below:

The depolarization _____ spreads quickly over both atria causing them to contract.

107. This depolarization wave is *not* conducted by the fibrous layer which separates the atria from the ventricles of the heart. Instead the wave is passed to the ventricles via the atrio-ventricular (A-V) bundle.

The tissue of the A-V bundle is cardiac muscle tissue modified to provide a high conduction rate for

the _____ wave.

108. A septum, or partition, separates the right and

_____ ventricles.

109. The A-V _____ originates at the atrio-ventricular node and passes along this septum.

110. The atrial depolarization wave is picked up at the A-V node and carried via the A-V bundle to the apex of the heart from which it spreads *upward*

over the _____.

bundle

111. A complete or partial block may occur in the bundle tissue. Such a block prevents or modifies the

passage of the _____ wave from the atria to the ventricles.

ventricles

112. Depending on the degree of A-V block, the atria

and _____ will have different rates of rhythmic contraction.

depolarization

113. The *contraction* of the heart muscle follows the same order as *depolarization*. The contraction begins towards the upper (base) portion of the heart.

The upper chambers, or _____, contract first.

ventricles

114. Atrial contraction forces additional _____ into the ventricles.

atria

115. Contraction of the _____ begins at the bottom (apex) of the heart and spreads toward the top of the ventricles.

blood

116. Vessels carrying blood away from the heart are called arteries. Ventricular contraction forces

blood into the aorta and the pulmonary _____.

ventricles

117. The valves of the heart are passive structures; that is, they open or close in response to differences in

_____.

artery

118. The illustration on the next page is a functional diagram of the heart. Refer to it and complete the next few frames.

pressure

113

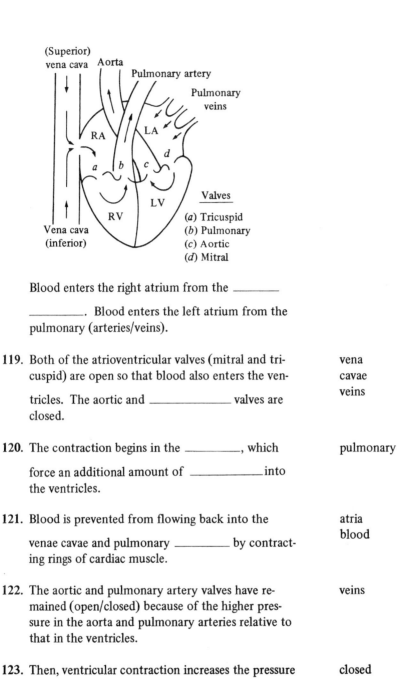

(Superior)
vena cava   Aorta
        Pulmonary artery
                Pulmonary
                veins

RA   LA

a b c d

Valves

RV   LV

Vena cava
(inferior)

(a) Tricuspid
(b) Pulmonary
(c) Aortic
(d) Mitral

Blood enters the right atrium from the _____

_____. Blood enters the left atrium from the
pulmonary (arteries/veins).

119. Both of the atrioventricular valves (mitral and tri-   vena
cuspid) are open so that blood also enters the ven-   cavae
                                                           veins
tricles. The aortic and _____ valves are
closed.

120. The contraction begins in the _____, which   pulmonary
force an additional amount of _____ into
the ventricles.

121. Blood is prevented from flowing back into the   atria
                                                             blood
venae cavae and pulmonary _____ by contract-
ing rings of cardiac muscle.

122. The aortic and pulmonary artery valves have re-   veins
mained (open/closed) because of the higher pres-
sure in the aorta and pulmonary arteries relative to
that in the ventricles.

123. Then, ventricular contraction increases the pressure   closed
within the _____.

114

124. When ventricular pressures become greater than atrial pressures, the A-V valves (mitral and tricuspid) close. What function does this serve?

ventricules

125. As ventricular contraction proceeds, the ventricular pressures (rise/fall/remain the same).

Closure prevents ventricular blood from entering the atria

126. When the ventricular pressures surpass aortic and pulmonary artery pressures the aortic and pulmonary valves (open/close).

rise

127. When these valves open, blood is forced into both the systemic and the _____ circulations.

open

128. After the blood leaves the ventricles the ventricular pressures (rise/fall) and the aortic and pulmonary valves (close/open).

pulmonary

129. As ventricular pressures continue to drop, the atrioventricular valves open, and again the ventricles (fill/empty).

fall
close

130. The contraction phase is called systole and lasts for about 0.3 second. Diastole is about 0.5 second long. It is the opposite of the contraction phase; that is, this is the _____ phase.

fill

131. The contraction phase is called _____ and the relaxation phase is called _____.

relaxation

132. What is the approximate duration of a complete cycle?

systole
diastole

133. One cycle every 0.8 second equals 60/0.8 or _____ cycles (beats) per minute.

0.8 second

134. An increase in heart rate (e.g., during exercise) is primarily at the expense of the relaxation phase or _____.

75

135. In other words, during exercise the heart rests for a (longer/shorter) time each cycle.

diastole

136. The major sounds of the heart beat occur with the closing of the valves. The first sound is coincident with closure of the atrioventricular _____ and sounds like "lub."

shorter

137. The second sound arises during the closing of the aortic and pulmonary _____ and sounds like "dup."

valves

138. Due to the relatively longer _____ (relaxation) phase, the overall cyclic sounds are "lub-dup" (pause), "lub-dup" (pause), "lub-dup" (pause), etc.

valves

139. Each ventricle normally ejects about 70 ml of blood during systole. This volume is called the *stroke volume.*

The output of one ventricle (cardiac output) during one minute of normal beating equals the volume ejected per beat (_____ml) times the number of beats (how many?) per minute.

diastolic

140. Or, stated another way, cardiac output equals stroke _____ times heart _____.

70
75

141. Calculate cardiac output from the following: 70 ml/beat X 75 beats/ min =

volume, rate

142. The large arteries are elastic and distend to accommodate the volume of blood ejected during _____ (phase).

5250 ml/min

143. During diastole, when no blood enters the arteries, the elastic recoil of the arteries maintains blood flow to the capillaries. The veins return the blood to the heart. Thus blood flow in the blood vessels does not cease during diastole due to this distension and recoil of the arteries. The flow is pulsatile in the (arteries/veins)

systole

144. Under normal circumstances the left ventricle develops a pressure of about 120 mm Hg during systole. This pressure falls to the pressure level of the thorax (about 0 mm Hg) during the relaxation

phase, or _____.

arteries

145. The pressure in the *aorta,* however, falls only to about 80 mm Hg due to closure of the aortic valve

and the elastic recoil of the _____.

diastole

146. The pressures indicated above are relative to the atmospheric pressure outside the body. For example, if the outside pressure were 760 mm Hg then the "true" thorax pressure would also be 760 mm Hg. The relative pressure (inside-outside) equals 0 mm Hg. Similarly, "true" systolic pressure would equal 880 mm Hg, and relative systolic pressure would equal 880 mm Hg minus the "true" thorax

pressure, giving _____ mm Hg.

aorta (arteries)

147. Blood pressure can be estimated with an inflatable cuff connected to a mercury manometer (sphygmomanometer). These pressures are recorded as $\frac{120}{80}$. The top number represents the systolic pressure

and the lower number represents the _____ pressure.

120 mm Hg

diastolic

NOTE: The cuff around the arm is inflated, which closes off arterial flow. The pressure is then reduced in the cuff until arterial flow just begins. This is determined by listening for the turbulent flow of blood past the cuff with a stethoscope. At this point, the systolic pressure is recorded from the manometer. Diastolic pressure is determined from the change or disappearance of the flow sound as the cuff pressure is further reduced to allow the flow of blood without restriction.

148. Flow through the large veins near the heart shows some pulsation due to reflection of the pressure changes within the upper heart chambers or _____.

149. Sounds other than the normal heart sounds are called *murmurs* and may arise from the turbulent flow of blood through impaired *valves.* These abnormal sounds or _____ are termed diastolic or systolic, depending on their time of occurrence in the cardiac cycle.

atria

150. *Stenosis* is a narrowing of a valve orifice. This kind of valve impairment can increase the turbulence of blood flow through the valves and thus can give rise to a _____.

murmurs

151. The depolarization of the cardiac muscle follows a regular pattern that may be recorded electrically from leads attached to the body. The recording of the electrical changes occurring during the cardiac cycle is abbreviated ECG. The letters stand for

electro _____ gram.

murmur

152. Not only the electrical behavior of the heart but also the location of the recording leads determine the particular pattern obtained in an

_____.

electrocardiagram
(sometimes you will
see EKG which
means the same
thing)

153. For this latter reason the positions of the leads have been standardized. The leads may be connected to the arms, legs, or chest. Usually several combinations of leads are utilized to obtain an overall picture.

electrocardiogram

A sample ECG is shown on the following page.

With each heart beat, one series of waves occurs. A single series of waves in the ECG are lettered *P*,

___, ___, ___, and ___.

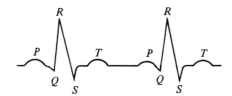

154. The first or *P*-wave is coincident with atrial depolarization; that is, the *P*-wave is recorded as the
depolarization wave spreads from the S-A node

over the _____ .

Q, R, S, and *T*

155. Thus we say that the *P*-wave is coincident with

_____ depolarization.

atria

156. The impulse spreads across the atria and down the
A-V bundle tissue during the *P-Q* interval (beginning of *P*-wave to *Q*-wave).

atrial

157. During the *P-Q* interval, the impulse spreads across

the _____ and down the A-V _____ tissue.

158. The *Q-R-S* complex arises during ventricular depolarization. During this same time, repolarization

begins in the _____ .

atria, bundle

159. Thus the *Q-R-S* complex arises during ventricular

_____ and atrial

_____ .

atria

160. The *T*-wave, which follows depolarization (and
contraction) of the ventricles, is related to re-

polarization of the _____ .

depolarization
repolarization

161. Thus the *T*-wave is coincident with ventricular

_____ .

ventricles

119

162. To review, the *P*-wave records _____
_____. Then, during the *P-Q*
interval the impulse has spread across the _____
and down the A-V _____ tissue.

repolarization

163. The *Q-R-S* complex occurs during ventricular
_____ and atrial
_____.

atrial
depolarization
atria
bundle

164. Finally, the *T*-wave records ventricular
_____.

depolarization
repolarization

165. It should be noted that depolarization precedes
contraction. Therefore, the *Q-R-S* complex occurs
at the beginning of _____ contrac-
tion.

repolarization

166. A *prolongation* of the *P-R* interval would indicate
that the time required for impulse conduction
through the bundle is (increased/decreased).

ventricular

167. An abnormally shaped _____ recording might
arise from an altered ventricular muscle following a
coronary thrombosis.

increased

168. Normally, heart muscle contracts in a definite pattern. It is possible, however, for different parts of
the heart muscle to _____ out of
phase; that is, uncoordinated contractions occur in
different parts of the _____.

Q-R-S

169. *Fibrillation* is the term used to describe these abnormal uncoordinated _____.

depolarize (contract)
heart

170. If the uncoordinated contractions occur in the
atria, it is called atrial _____.

contractions

120

171. Immediate cessation of blood flow results from ventricular _____.

        fibrillation

NOTE: Atrial fibrillation is not fatal but merely reduces the amount of ventricular filling during diastole. Ventricular fibrillation, however, is fatal unless suitable means (cardiac massage) are immediately used to maintain circulation.

172. Blood flow is fairly constant through the systemic and pulmonary circulation. Recall the equation relating blood flow to pressure and resistance:

$$\text{flow} = \frac{\text{blood pressure}}{\text{peripheral resistance}}$$

Thus, if the flow remains constant, an increase in peripheral resistance (PR) is accompanied by an increase in _____ _____.

        fibrillation

173. The degree of venous distention in part determines the amount of blood available to enter the heart (venous return) during the relaxation phase, known as _____.

        blood pressure

174. The amount of blood that the large veins hold is regulated by the *sympathetic nervous system.* Thus, vasomotor tone in the large veins is controlled by impulses from the _____ nervous system.

        diastole

175. So, if the veins are constricted, more blood is available to enter the ventricles and the stroke volume is (increased/decreased).

        sympathetic

176. Vasoconstriction of the large veins can partially compensate for a certain amount of blood loss by maintaining _____ return to the heart.

        increased

NOTE: The following diagram summarizes changes in aortic pressure (————), atrial pressure (· · · ·), left ventricular pressure (———), ventricular volume (——— ———), ECG and heart sounds (below) during the cardiac cycle.

121

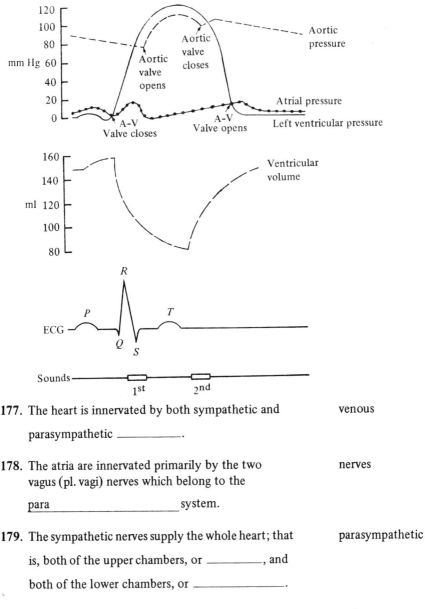

177. The heart is innervated by both sympathetic and parasympathetic _____.

    venous

178. The atria are innervated primarily by the two vagus (pl. vagi) nerves which belong to the para_____ system.

    nerves

179. The sympathetic nerves supply the whole heart; that is, both of the upper chambers, or _____, and both of the lower chambers, or _____.

    parasympathetic

180. The parasympathetic nerves primarily innervate the _____ while the sympathetic nerves supply the _____ heart. The vagi are nerves of the _____ system of the autonomic nervous system.

    atria
    ventricles

122

181. Impulses arriving over the vagus nerves cause the heart to slow down. Thus, the heart slows down when the _____ nerves are stimulated.

atria
whole
parasympathetic

182. On the other hand, sympathetic nerve action is just the opposite. So when the sympathetic nerves are stimulated, the heart rate (increases/decreases).

vagus

183. As previously mentioned, *venous return* determines blood flow from the heart, or cardiac _____.

increases

184. Blood flow from the heart or cardiac output is dependent on _____ _____.

output

185. Venous return is determined in part by the degree of *constriction* of the venous system.

So, one factor determining venous return is the degree of _____ of the venous system.

venous return

186. Another factor determining venous return is the volume of blood within the entire circulatory system.

Therefore, venous return also depends in part on the _____ of blood within the entire _____ system.

constriction

187. To summarize, the factors that determine the amount of venous return include the degree of _____ of the venous system and the blood _____ within the circulatory system.

volume
circulatory

188. The blood volume in turn is regulated at the *capillary* level and by the kidneys. Let's look at these one at a time.

constriction
volume

189. The movement of fluid into or out of the capillaries depends on three things. One is the hydrostatic pressure difference across the _____ wall.

190. Fluid movement also depends on the osmotic pressure difference of the fluid across this wall and the permeability of the _____ to the fluid.

capillary

191. The hydrostatic pressure difference across the _____ wall varies from one end of the capillary to the other. That is, from the _____ end of the capillary to the _____ end of the capillary.

wall

192. This is shown in the next figure: the normal interstitial fluid pressure (or tissue pressure, TP) is about 1 mm Hg.

capillary
arterial
venous

	Capillary			
Venous end	BP15	BP25	BP35	Arterial end
	TP1	TP1	TP1	

Study the figure. Providing that the capillary is permeable to the fluid, will the effect of the hydrostatic pressure difference be to force water into or out of the capillary?

193. The fluid to which the capillary wall is _____ consists primarily of water and dissolved salts.

out of

194. The capillary wall is relatively impermeable to plasma proteins. Hence, interstitial space contains very (much/little) protein from the plasma.

permeable

195. Thus the concentrations of protein on the two sides of the capillary membrane are much (different/the same).

little

196. This concentration difference of protein creates

an osmotic _____ difference of water

across the capillary _____.

different

197. Water (can/cannot) pass easily through the capillary wall. But, in contrast, the plasma proteins (can/cannot) pass easily across the capillary wall.

pressure
wall (membrane)

198. Inside the capillary the concentration of water is (lower/higher). Thus osmotic pressure tends to drive water (into/out of) the capillary.

can
cannot

NOTE: Both the osmotic pressure difference and the hydrostatic pressure difference may be expressed in mm Hg. The osmotic pressure due to the presence of proteins is often called the colloid osmotic pressure (COP). These driving forces for water movement across the capillary wall are summarized in the next figure.

Capillary

Venous end	BP 15	BP 25	BP 35	Arterial end
	COP 28	COP 28	COP 28	

TP 1	TP 1
COP 4	COP 4

199. Use the illustration to complete the next few frames. The effect of blood pressure (hydrostatic pressure) is to force water (into/out of) the capillary.

lower
into

200. On the other hand, COP tends to retain water

_____ the capillary.

out of

201. It may therefore be seen that at the arterial end the *net* effect of the driving forces is to move water

_____ _____ the capillary.

in

202. At the venous end, the net effect is to move water

_____ the capillary.

out of

125

203. An increase in the capillary blood pressure (hydro-static pressure) increases the movement of

_____ from the capillary.

into

204. And a decrease in COP (reflecting a lower plasma protein concentration) (increases/decreases) water loss from the capillary.

water

205. In addition to blood capillaries, the interstitial spaces are also served by *lymphatic capillaries.* The lymphatic capillaries empty into the lymphatic ducts which connect with the venous system.

increases

206. The lymphatic ducts connect with the venous sys-

tem. The lymphatic _____ empty into the lymphatic ducts.

207. About 10% of the fluid leaving the blood capillaries

enters the _____ capillaries and returns to the venous system via the lymph ducts.

capillaries

208. *Edema* refers to the accumulation of fluid outside the capillaries. This accumulation of fluid outside

the capillaries is called _____.

lymphatic

209. In addition to the removal of water, the lymph capillaries remove protein and other large particles which may have leaked into the interstitial space.

edema

210. Most of the large thoracic and neck arteries con-tain special nerve endings called pressoreceptors. Stretching of one of these arteries, due to increas-ing pressure, stimulates the special nerve endings in

the arteries called _____.

211. The walls of the aortic arch and of the internal carotid arteries (carotid sinus area) are sensitive to changes of pressure because they contain a large

number of _____.

pressoreceptors

126

212. The medulla is the part of the CNS which receives the nerve impulses from these _____.

pressoreceptors

213. Pressoreceptor impulses inhibit the sympathetic center in the medulla and excite the

_____ center.

pressoreceptors

214. Pressoreceptor impulses inhibit the _____ center in the medulla and excite the

_____ center.

parasympathetic

215. Thus, when the pressoreceptors are stimulated, *sympathetic stimulation* to the heart and blood vessels is (increased/decreased).

sympathetic
parasympathetic

216. Is blood pressure increased or decreased by pressoreceptor stimulation?

decreased

217. Decreased sympathetic stimulation leads to a decreased cardiac rate, decreased strength of contraction and vasodilation in the peripheral circulatory system. And, in addition, increased *parasympathetic* stimulation tends to (decrease/increase) the heart rate.

decreased

218. Thus, a decrease in blood pressure results from (increasing/decreasing) heart rate and from vasodilation of the _____ _____.

decrease

219. Thus, a decrease in blood pressure results from

_____ heart rate and _____ of the blood vessels.

decreasing
blood vessels

220. Due to reduced blood pressure, the activity of the pressoreceptors (decreases/increases).

slowing (decreasing)
vasodilation

127

221. The *pressoreceptor reflex* just described is important during changes in body position. This reflex
maintains blood pressure and blood flow to the
head when standing up from a lying position.

The reflex that maintains blood pressure during

changes in body position is called the _____

_____.

decreases

pressoreceptor
reflex

You have now completed Section IV of Human Physiology. In this unit you
covered the functions and interrelations of the important structures of the circulatory system. In Section V we will discuss the physiology of respiration. We suggest a short break before continuing.

SECTION V

RESPIRATION

Respiration comprises (1) external respiration, which includes the exchange of gases in the alveoli of the lungs, breathing movements which renew the air in the lungs, and the mechanisms regulating these movements; (2) the transport of oxygen and carbon dioxide by the blood; (3) internal respiration, or the utilization of oxygen at the cellular level.

1. Breathing serves to maintain a relatively constant composition of gases in the air sacs or *alveoli* of the lungs. It does this by adding _____ (O_2) from the atmosphere and expelling _____

   _____ (CO_2) into the atmosphere.

2. During breathing water vapor is also lost to the

   _____.

3. Let's see how this occurs. As blood passes through the alveoli, it takes oxygen from the alveolar air

   and gives up carbon _____.

4. Although the relative proportions are different, the alveoli of the lungs contain the same gases as are

   present in the _____.

oxygen
carbon
dioxide

atmosphere

dioxide

129

5. That is, the alveoli contain the same gases present in the atmosphere, but/and in (different/the same) proportions.

atmosphere

6. The average composition of *alveolar gas* (Alv.), *inspired air* (Insp.), and *expired air* (Exp.) are given in the following table.

different

RESPIRATORY GAS COMPOSITION

(Partial pressures are given in mm Hg. Percentage composition given in ( )'s. The Total pressure equals 760 mm Hg.)

	O_2	CO_2	N_2	H_2O
Insp.	158 (20.4)	0.3 (.04)	596 (78.5)	variable
Alv.	104 (13.7)	40 (5.2)	569 (74.9)	47 (6.2)
Exp.	118 (15.5)	27 (3.5)	568 (74.8)	47 (6.2)

The variables used to describe changes in a gas are as follows:

P = pressure
V = volume
T = temperature (absolute)
n = number of moles
R = the gas constant (0.0821 liter atm/deg/mole)

The Gas Law relates these variables by the algebraic expression $PV = nRT$. By transformation, this formula is: (Complete the formula.)

$$P = \frac{nRT}{\underline{\quad ? \quad}}$$

7. It may be seen from the Gas Law that, when n and T are constant, an increase in pressure occurs with a(n) (increase/decrease) in volume.

V

130

8. Suppose instead that the volume and number of moles are held constant. Then an increase in temperature results in a(n) (increase/decrease) in pressure.

decrease

9. Suppose a given volume (constant V) contains a mixture of gases (1, 2, 3) at constant T. The Gas Law may be written for each gas as follows:

increase

$$P_1 V = n_1 RT$$
$$P_2 V = n_2 RT$$
$$P_3 V = \underline{\hspace{2cm}}$$

10. In the total volume, $n_1 + n_2 + n_3$ equals the total number of _____ of gas.

$n_3 RT$

11. $P_1 + P_2 + P_3$ equals the total _____ existing in the total volume.

moles

12. P_1, P_2, and P_3 are called the *partial* _____ of gases 1, 2, and 3.

pressure

NOTE: The partial pressure of a gas is directly proportional to the number of moles of that gas. The movement of a gas occurs from a region of higher pressure to one of lower pressure. In a mixture of gases each gas exerts a partial pressure proportional to the concentration of that gas in the mixture. In such a mixture each gas will tend to move from a region of higher to a region of lower partial pressure of that gas.

13. An understanding of the partial pressure concept is essential to the description of oxygen and carbon dioxide movements between the lungs and the metabolizing cells of the body. Suppose a container holds a mixture of nitrogen and oxygen. Part of the pressure of the mixture will be due to the nitrogen and part will be due to the _____.

pressures

14. If the molar ratio of nitrogen to oxygen is 3 to 2, what part of the total pressure is attributable only to the nitrogen?

oxygen

15. So the partial pressure of the N_2 is 3/5 of the

_____ pressure.

3/5

16. Let us go on to another example. A gas mixture with a total pressure of 600 mm Hg contains twice as much O_2 as N_2 ($nO_2 = 2nN_2$). State the partial pressure of N_2 (PN_2) as a fraction of the total pressure (600 mm Hg).

total

17. What, then, is the *partial pressure* of N_2 expressed in mm Hg?

1/3 of total pressure

18. An equation often facilitates partial pressure calculations. Follow this one, beginning with

$PN_2 = 200$ mm Hg

$$\frac{PO_2 V}{PN_2 V} = \frac{nO_2 RT}{nN_2 RT}$$

Notice that the V and RT terms cancel and that we are left with

$$\frac{PO_2}{PN_2} = ?$$

19. $\dfrac{PO_2}{PN_2} = \dfrac{nO_2}{nN_2} = \dfrac{2}{1}$; therefore $PO_2 = 2PN_2$

$\dfrac{nO_2}{nN_2}$

$$PO_2 + PN_2 = 600 \text{ mm Hg}$$

$$2PN_2 + PN_2 = 600 \text{ mm Hg}$$

$$3PN_2 = 600 \text{ mm Hg}$$

Thus, $PN_2 = $ ____ mm Hg

NOTE: When calculating the partial pressure of a gas, all gases in the mixture must be considered, including the vapor pressure of water, if water is present. This becomes important when calculating the partial pressures of the gases in alveolar air, which is saturated with water vapor. The partial pressure of water vapor depends on temperature. At body temperature (37°C) vapor pressure is 47 mm Hg.

20. Nitrogen (N_2) throughout the body is equilibrated with atmospheric nitrogen and is not utilized in metabolism by the body. The difference in the partial pressures of N_2 in inspired air and expired air arises from the inclusion in the expired air of

    water _____. Percentage composition is given by the *partial* pressure of a gas divided by the *total* _____ of the mixture, times 100.

    200

21. Question:

    $$\frac{PO_2}{P_{tot.}} \times 100 = \% \text{ of } \underline{\hspace{1cm}} \text{ (what gas?)}$$

    vapor pressure

22. When a gas mixture is in contact with a liquid (e.g., water or plasma), the partial pressures of the gases approach an equilibrium between the gas and liquid phases. That is, the partial pressures of gases dissolved in the liquid phase approach in the

    _____ phase.

    O_2

23. The amount of a gas that will dissolve in water depends on the nature of the particular gas, the temperature, and the partial _____ of that gas.

    gas

24. The concentration of a gas dissolved in the liquid phase may be determined as in the following example:

    $$\text{conc. } O_2 = \alpha O_2 \times PO_2$$

    where α is the solubility coefficient for a gas in a particular liquid at a given temperature.

    $$\alpha O_2 \text{ in water at } 0°C = \frac{0.003 \text{ ml } O_2}{100 \text{ ml water/mm Hg}}$$

    Thus, conc. CO_2 = _____ $\times PCO_2$

    $$\alpha CO_2 = \frac{0.075 \text{ ml } CO_2}{100 \text{ ml water/mm Hg}}$$

    pressure

133

25. Example: Determine the concentration of oxygen in solution, using information from the following diagram.

αCO_2

Concentration of O_2 = αO_2 × PO_2

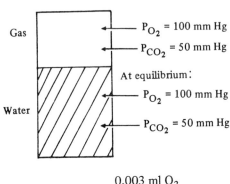

Gas
P_{O_2} = 100 mm Hg
P_{CO_2} = 50 mm Hg

At equilibrium:
P_{O_2} = 100 mm Hg

Water
P_{CO_2} = 50 mm Hg

$$\alpha O_2 = \frac{0.003 \text{ ml } O_2}{100 \text{ ml water/mm Hg}}$$

Now let's substitute values from the diagram above.

$$\text{conc. } O_2 = \frac{0.003 \text{ ml } O_2}{100 \text{ ml water/mm Hg}} \times 100 \text{ mm Hg } O_2$$

Solving for conc. O_2 we get:

$$\frac{0.3 \text{ ml } O_2}{100 \text{ ml water}} = \underline{\hspace{2cm}} \text{ volumes per cent}$$

26. Now calculate the concentration of CO_2 in the above example.

0.3

27. The diffusion of a gas, either in the gas phase or dissolved in a liquid, occurs from a region of higher

_____ pressure to a region of lower

_____ pressure of that gas.

conc. CO_2
= 50 × 0.075
= 3.8 vol %

28. The diffusion of O_2 and CO_2 across the alveolar walls of the lungs occurs from regions of

_____ partial pressures to regions of

_____ partial pressures of these gases.

partial
partial

134

29. As indicated in the figure below, venous blood
    enting the lungs comes into contact with the

    membranes of the _____.

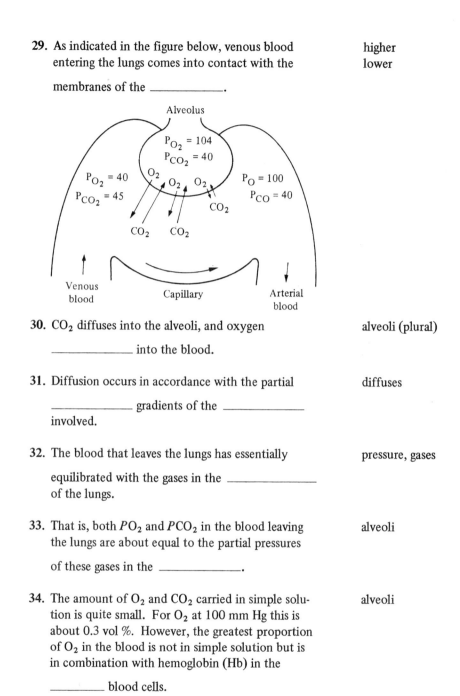

30. CO_2 diffuses into the alveoli, and oxygen

    _____ into the blood.

31. Diffusion occurs in accordance with the partial

    _____ gradients of the _____
    involved.

32. The blood that leaves the lungs has essentially

    equilibrated with the gases in the _____
    of the lungs.

33. That is, both PO_2 and PCO_2 in the blood leaving
    the lungs are about equal to the partial pressures

    of these gases in the _____.

34. The amount of O_2 and CO_2 carried in simple solu-
    tion is quite small. For O_2 at 100 mm Hg this is
    about 0.3 vol %. However, the greatest proportion
    of O_2 in the blood is not in simple solution but is
    in combination with hemoglobin (Hb) in the

    _____ blood cells.

higher
lower

alveoli (plural)

diffuses

pressure, gases

alveoli

alveoli

35. Dissolved oxygen passes into the red blood cells and forms a loosely bound compound called oxy-hemoglobin (HbO_2).

    Oxygen combines loosely with hemoglobin in the

    red blood cells to form _____.

red

36. The combining of oxygen and hemoglobin may be expressed as:

    $$Hb + \underline{} \rightarrow HbO_2$$

oxyhemoglobin

37. The amount of oxygen combining with hemoglobin (the per cent saturation of oxygen with Hb) de-

    pends on the partial pressure of _____ in the blood.

O_2

38. This relation is shown in the next graph:

oxygen

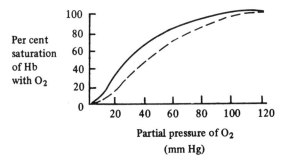

Per cent saturation of Hb with O_2

Partial pressure of O_2
(mm Hg)

    The solid line on the graph shows that as the PO_2 increases, the per cent of the hemoglobin that will combine with oxygen (increases/decreases).

39. The dotted line shows an effect of increased PCO_2

    on the combination of _____ and

    _____.

increases

40. Increased PCO_2 (increases/decreases) the ability of hemoglobin to combine with oxygen.

oxygen
hemoglobin (Hb)
(either order)

41. So, for a given PO_2 as the PCO_2 is increased, the per cent saturation of hemoglobin with O_2 will (increase/decrease).

decreases

42. As PCO_2 is decreased, will more or less O_2 combine with Hb?

decrease

136

43. Carbon dioxide is transported in the blood in four forms: about 5% is dissolved CO_2 and carbonic acid, 30% is carbamino compounds, 65% is bicarbonate ions. Which form would you expect to be most prevalent in blood?

more

44. When carbon dioxide is dissolved in blood, carbonic acid is formed. Complete the expression.

(carbonic acid) $H_2CO_3 \leftrightharpoons H_2O + \underline{\hspace{1cm}}$

bicarbonate ions

45. When carbon dioxide is dissolved in blood, it combines with water to form $\underline{\hspace{2cm}}$ $\underline{\hspace{1.5cm}}$.

CO_2

46. The formation of carbonic acid from dissolved CO_2 is accelerated by the enzyme *carbonic anhydrase* which is present in the red blood cell.

Carbonic acid formation from dissolved CO_2 is accelerated by an enzyme known as carbonic

$\underline{\hspace{3cm}}$.

carbonic acid

47. The carbonic acid then *dissociates* into *hydrogen* and *bicarbonate* ions. Complete the expression.

$H_2CO_3 \leftrightharpoons \underline{\hspace{1cm}} + HCO_3^-$ (bicarbonate ions)

anhydrase

48. In addition to forming carbonic acid, carbon dioxide also combines loosely with hemoglobin and plasma proteins to form *carbamino* compounds ($HbCO_2$). These compounds involving CO_2 and protein are called $\underline{\hspace{2cm}}$ compounds.

H^+ or (hydrogen ions

49. Carbamino compounds consist of $\underline{\hspace{1cm}}$ and plasma [proteins or hemoglobin (Hb)]. The reactions of CO_2 in blood are summarized in the following diagram:

carbamino

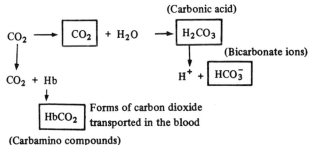

(Carbonic acid)

$CO_2 \rightarrow \boxed{CO_2} + H_2O \rightarrow \boxed{H_2CO_3}$

(Bicarbonate ions)

$CO_2 + Hb$

$H^+ + \boxed{HCO_3^-}$

$\boxed{HbCO_2}$ Forms of carbon dioxide transported in the blood

(Carbamino compounds)

50. The rate at which O_2 is supplied to the tissue capillaries depends on the amount of _____ in the blood (combined with Hb) and the rate at which the heart pumps the _____ to the tissues.

CO_2

51. What two factors determine the rate at which O_2 is supplied to the tissue capillaries?

O_2
blood

52. The transfer of oxygen and carbon dioxide across the capillary walls in the systemic circulation is the reverse of the transfers occurring in the pulmonary circulation. The diagram below illustrates the transfer of O_2 and CO_2 between·tissue and _____.

1. amount of O_2 in the blood
2. rate at which the heart pumps blood to the tissues

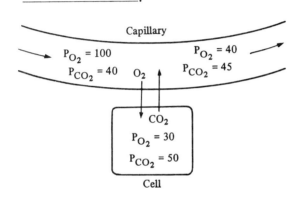

NOTE: A review of the anatomy of the chest should be made with special attention to the respiratory passageways (trachea, bronchii, etc.), the rib cage, the diaphragm, the lungs, and the intrapleural space (pleural cavity).

53. The *pleural membranes,* which line the intrapleural space, absorb *gases* and *fluids* to a point where there is no real intrapleural space at all. That is, the inner pleural membrane (which is on contact with the lungs) is normally in contact with the

outer pleural _____, which is in contact with the chest wall.

54. The pressure in the potential intrapleural "space" is below atmospheric _____.

55. This reduced pressure helps to keep the lungs expanded closely against the _____ wall.

56. The lungs are elastic and would collapse if the _____ "space" were opened to atmospheric pressure.

57. The lungs increase and decrease in volume by following the movements of the rib cage and diaphragm. *Inspiration* is brought about primarily by the diaphragm and by the *external intercostal muscles.*

Inspiration occurs primarily through the work of

the _____ and the external

_____ muscles.

58. Thus, inspiration occurs when the external intercostals move the rib cage upward and outward. This action (increases/decreases) the volume of the thorax.

59. The muscles that increase the volume of the thorax

by moving the rib cage are the _____

_____.

60. The action of the diaphragm is illustrated in the next figure:

capillaries

membrane

pressure

chest

intrapleural

diaphragm
intercostal

increases

external
intercostals

139

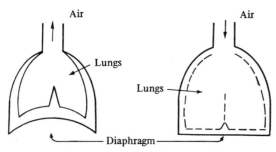

Air	Air
Lungs	Lungs

(a) Relaxed (b) Contracted
(external intercostals and diaphragm) (external intercostals and diaphragm)

Diaphragm

In the illustration you can see that contraction of
the diaphragm (increases/decreases) the lung volume.

61. Normally *expiration* is accomplished by a simple   increases
    relaxation of the muscles that caused the previous

    _____.

62. When this relaxation occurs the elastic properties   inspiration
    of the chest and lungs (reduce/increase) the
    thoracic volume.

63. A *forced* expiration involves, in addition, the   reduce
    contraction of other muscles that reduce the

    _____ volume.

64. The total adult lung volume after a full inspiration   thoracic
    is about 6 liters. After normal expiration, about
    2.4 liters of air still remain in the lungs.

65. The total adult lung volume is about _____

    liters; after normal expiration about _____
    liters remain in the lungs.

66. After a *forced* maximum expiration, the volume of   6
    air remaining is termed the *residual volume.* This   2.4
    is about one-half the amount that remains in the
    lungs following a normal expiration. Residual

    volume, then, is about _____.

140

67. The amount of air left in the lungs after a forced maximum expiration is called the _____ _____.

1.2 liters

68. That volume of air that can be forcefully expired after taking a *full* breath (maximum inspiration) is termed the *vital capacity*. This volume varies with a person's age and the condition of his lungs. After taking a full breath, an average individual can forcefully expire all but about 1.2 liters volume. The volume that can be expired is called

_____ _____.

residual volume

69. *Tidal volume* is that volume of air which a person normally *inspires* and _____.

vital capacity

70. The volume of air normally inspired and expired is the _____ _____. These divisions of the total lung volume are shown below:

expires

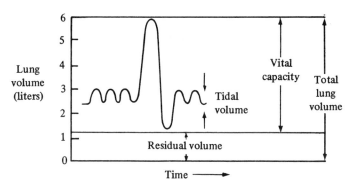

The volume of all the respiratory passages (excluding the alveoli) is called *dead space.*

71. Thus, with each breath, the amount of *fresh* air that enters the alveoli is equal to the tidal volume *less* the volume of the dead _____.

tidal volume

72. If the tidal volume becomes much smaller than the dead space volume no fresh air will reach the

   _____.

   space

73. When this happens, gas exchange between the alveoli and pulmonary blood (decreases/increases).

   alveoli

74. Nervous pathways originating in the *medulla* and *pons* of the brain control rhythmic breathing. The diagram below illustrates the factors affecting breathing.

   decreases

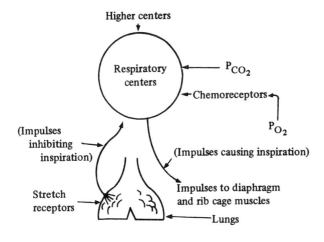

75. Thus, the medulla and pons contain the

   _____ centers of the brain.

76. Blood levels of O_2 and CO_2 influence the action of the _____ centers.

   respiratory

77. Thus, we can say that the respiratory centers located in the medulla and pons are affected by

   blood levels of _____ and _____. A change in PCO_2 is the primary agent that acts on the respiratory centers to change respiratory rate.

   respiratory

78. The respiratory centers are also responsive to impulses from higher centers of the brain (as in speaking) and to impulses arriving from *stretch receptors* in the lungs.

O_2, CO_2

The respiratory centers are influenced both by

impulses from _____ _____ of the

brain and impulses from _____

_____ in the lungs.

79. An increase in blood CO_2 stimulates respiration primarily by its direct effect on the

_____ _____.

higher centers
stretch
receptors

80. What would be the effect of low blood CO_2 (increased or decreased respiration)?

respiratory centers

81. Located in the aorta, the carotid arteries and the pulmonary artery are chemoreceptors that are sensitive to a large decrease in PO_2.

decreased respiration

82. Thus, a large decrease in PO_2 increases impulses

from the O_2 _____.

83. There, chemoreceptor impulses are carried to the respiratory centers and lead to a(n) (increase/ decrease) in breathing rate.

chemoreceptors

84. Inflation of the lungs during inspiration stimulates the *stretch receptors* of the lungs. Stretch receptor impulses inhibit the respiratory center which is causing (inspiration/expiration).

increase

85. Thus, the inspiratory part of respiration is inhibited

by _____ _____ impulses to the
brain.

inspiration

86. After the muscles of inspiration are inhibited, (inspiration/expiration) occurs.

stretch receptor

87. So you can see that normal cyclic breathing is, in part, dependent on the _____ _____ reflex (Hering-Breuer reflex).

expiration

88. During speech, higher centers of the brain take part in the control of breathing. Thus, higher centers of the brain take part in the control of respiratory movements while a person is _____ .

stretch receptor

89. The lungs play a major role in the regulation of the hydrogen ion concentration of the blood. The acidity or alkalinity of the blood depends on the H$^+$ (hydrogen ion) concentration of the _____ .

speaking

90. The H$^+$ concentration is usually expressed as pH, which indicates the blood's _____ or _____ .

blood

91. pH is equal to the logarithm of 1/H$^+$, or (complete the expression):

$$\underline{\hspace{2cm}} = \log \frac{1}{H^+}$$

acidity
alkalinity

$$pH = \left[\log \frac{1}{H^+} \right]$$

NOTE: The definition and properties of logarithms are given below as an aid to understanding pH and buffers.

LOGARITHMS: A number (b) raised to a power (p) gives an answer (a). This may be expressed as:

$$bP = a$$

For example,

$$10^{-1} = 0.1$$
$$2^3 = 8$$
$$8^2 = 64$$

This relation may also be expressed in logarithmic fashion:

$$\log_{(b)} a = p$$

which states that the logarithm to the base b of a equals p. The logarithm of a, then, is the power (p) to which b must be raised to equal a. Although any base (b) *may be used, the number* 10 *is in common use and is usually implied in the abbreviation "log." With respect to the base* 10, *the following relations hold:*

$$10^p = a$$
$$10^{-1} = 0.1$$
$$10^0 = 1$$
$$10^1 = 10$$
$$10^2 = 100, \text{ etc.}$$

or,

$$\log a = p$$
$$\log 0.1 = -1$$
$$\log 1 = 0$$
$$\log 10 = 1$$
$$\log 100 = 2, \text{ etc.}$$

When the number (a) *is between* 1 *and* 10, *the log of* a *will lie between* 0 *and* 1. *If* a *is between* 10 *and* 100, *its logarithm will lie between* 1 *and* 2. *For example,*

$$\log 8 = 0.9031$$
$$\log 35 = 1.5441$$
$$\log 3.5 = 0.5441$$

The number to the left of the decimal point (called the characteristic) of the logarithm is determined by the position of a (*between* 1 *and* 10, *between* 10 *and* 100 *etc.*). *The number to the right of the decimal point (called the mantissa) is determined from a table of logarithms. The following properties are associated with logarithms:*

$$\log x + \log y = \log (xy)$$
$$\log x - \log y = \log (x/y)$$
$$c \log x = \log x^c$$

92. You'll recall that the following compounds form when CO_2 enters blood.

$$CO_2 + H_2O \rightarrow H_2CO_3 \text{ (carbonic acid)}$$
$$H_2CO_3 \rightarrow HCO_3^- + H^+ \text{ (bicarbonate ions +}$$
$$\text{hydrogen ions)}$$

The HCO_3^- and H_2CO_3 pair act as a buffer, that is, the

_____ _____ and _____

_____ pair act as a buffer.

93. A buffer tends to prevent large changes in the

hydrogen ion concentration (or ____) of the blood.

bicarbonate ions
carbonic acid

145

94. The *pH* of the blood is related to the *relative* amounts of HCO_3^- and H_2CO_3 in the blood. These compounds are a _____ pair.

pH

buffer

NOTE: The relation of pH to HCO_3^- and H_2CO_3 is given below as an aid to understanding.

BUFFER EQUATION: The equilibrium relation of carbonic acid dissociation,

$$H_2CO_3 \rightarrow H^+ + HCO_3^-$$

can be expressed as

$$\frac{H^+ \times HCO_3^-}{H_2CO_3} = K$$

in which K is called the equilibrium constant. This equation states that the product of the hydrogen ion concentration and the bicarbonate ion concentration divided by the carbonic acid concentration is a constant at equilibrium. This equation may be solved for H^+:

$$H^+ = K \times \frac{H_2CO_3}{HCO_3^-}$$

and may be rewritten as

$$\frac{1}{H^+} = \frac{1}{K} \times \frac{HCO_3^-}{H_2CO_3}$$

Taking logarithms to the base 10 of each side of this equation gives

$$\log \frac{1}{H^+} = \log \frac{1}{K} + \log \frac{HCO_3^-}{H_2CO_3}$$

The log of $1/H^+$ is called pH; log of $1/K$ is called pK. Then,

$$pH = pK + \log \frac{HCO_3^-}{H_2CO_3}$$

The neutral point on the pH scale is 7. Values below 7 are acidic; values above 7 are basic (alkalotic). Normal blood pH is about 7.4.

Plasma proteins, hemoglobin, $HPO_4^=$ and $H_2PO_4^-$ form other buffer systems found in the blood.

95. The amount of carbon dioxide dissolved in the blood determines the concentration of H_2CO_3, or _____ _____ in the blood.

146

96. The amount of dissolved CO_2 in the blood depends on the PCO_2 and the *solubility* coefficient of CO_2 in blood. So, by controlling blood PCO_2 (and thereby the H_2CO_3 concentration) respiration regulates the

   pH, or _____ _____ _____ of blood.

   carbonic acid

97. Increasing the respiratory rate decreases the alveolar PCO_2 and as a result (increases/decreases) blood PCO_2 and H_2CO_3.

   hydrogen
   ion concentration

98. What effect does holding your breath have on alveolar PCO_2?

   decreases

99. An increased PCO_2 in the alveoli leads to more dissolved CO_2 in the blood and thus the formation

   of more H_2CO_3, or _____ _____.

   increases PCO_2

100. If something changes the pH of blood (ingestion of acid or alkali, production of acids by metabolism, etc.) the respiratory centers respond by changing the respiratory rate which returns the blood

   _____ toward a normal of 7.4.

   carbonic acid

101. An increase in blood pH is compensated by a respiratory rate which (increases/decreases).

   pH

102. Slowed respiration allows the build up in the blood of carbonic acid which (lowers/raises) the pH toward normal.

   decreases

103. A decreased blood pH is compensated by a respiratory rate that (increases/decreases).

   lowers

NOTE: Other blood pH adjustments are made by the kidney in its control of HCO_3^- excretion. (This will be explored more fully in the section on Renal Physiology.)

104. Here are some review frames on respiration. The ideal gas law relates number of moles, temperature,

   volume, and _____.

   increases

147

105. At constant volume and temperature the partial pressure of a gas is directly proportional to the number of _____ of that gas.

pressure

106. The amount of gas that will dissolve in water depends on: the nature of that gas; the temperature; and its _____ _____.

moles

107. Blood leaving the lungs has equilibrated with the *gases* in the _____.

partial pressure

108. The greatest proportion of O_2 in the blood is in combination with _____.

alveoli

109. Carbon dioxide is transported in the blood in four forms: dissolved _____ _____ (CO_2), _____ _____ (H_2CO_3), _____ _____ (HCO_3^-), and _____ compounds such as $HbCO_2$.

hemoglobin

110. The amount of air left in the lungs after a *forced* expiration is called the _____ _____.

carbon dioxide
carbonic acid
bicarbonate ions
carbamino (com-pounds)

111. The volume of air normally inspired and expired is the _____ _____.

residual volume

112. Rhythmic breathing is controlled by nervous pathways originating in the _____ and _____.

tidal volume

113. A decreased blood pH is compensated by increasing the _____ _____.

pons, medulla

respiratory rate

148

Now you've completed Section V of Human Physiology. In this section you covered two phases of respiration, namely external respiration and transportation of oxygen and carbon dioxide by the blood. The utilization of oxygen at the cellular level is called internal respiration, which we have not taken up in this unit. Internal respiration can be covered more appropriately if you study biochemistry.

Before going on to Section VI, Renal Physiology, we recommend a short break.

SECTION VI

RENAL PHYSIOLOGY

The kidney is an organ of excretion and regulation. It removes the waste products of metabolism, such as nitrogen and sulfur, and by its excretory activity serves to regulate the plasma volume and water content of the body. The kidney also regulates the electrolyte balance of the organism by selectively excreting or conserving the ionic constituents of plasma. The kidney provides another means of maintaining a normal blood pH by controlling the bicarbonate level of the plasma.

1. The kidney is made up of a great number of functional units called *nephrons*. There are about a

   million nephrons in each human _____.

2. The illustration below is a functional representation of a nephron.   kidney

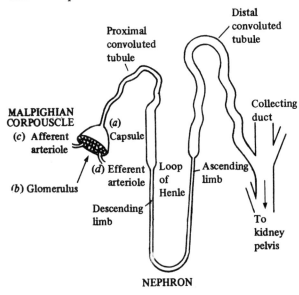

NEPHRON

150

A *nephron* consists of a Malpighian corpuscle and a
renal tubule which terminate in a _____

_____.

3. Refer to the figure again. The Malpighian corpus-   collecting
   cle consists of (a), a _____ and a   duct
   capillary tuft (b) called a _____.

4. Blood flows through the glomerulus and is regu-   capsule
   lated by *constriction* or *dilation* of its afferent (c)   glomerulus
   and efferent (d) arterioles. The renal tubule and
   collecting duct are well supplied with *capillaries*
   derived from the efferent arteriole of the

   _____.

5. The initial process of urine formation is *filtration*   glomerulus
   at the glomerulus. At the glomerulus, the first
   process in urine formation takes place. This is the

   process of _____.

6. Fluid is forced out of the *glomerular* capillary tuft,   filtration
   into the capsule and then into the renal tubule
   during the first process in urine formation, which

   is _____.

7. The fluid filtrate is derived directly from the blood   filtration
   and closely resembles the fluid part of blood,

   that is, the blood _____.

8. However, the glomerular filtrate differs from blood   plasma
   _____ in that the filtrate contains little or no
   protein.

9. Let's briefly review. The fluid formed at the be-   plasma
   ginning of the nephron is an *ultra*filtrate of plasma.
   It is formed by the process of glomerular

   _____.

151

NOTE: The rate *at which filtration occurs is called the glomerular filtration rate or GFR. The driving forces for glomerular filtration are the* hydrostatic pressure difference *and the* osmotic pressure difference *between glomerular capillary and renal tubule. These are the same forces that cause water movement in or out of capillaries in the tissues.*

10. Blood pressure is higher than renal tubular pressure. Therefore, the hydrostatic pressure difference tends to force fluid (into/out of) the glomerular capillaries.

    filtration

11. Now compare capillary blood protein content with the protein content of the *ultrafiltrate*. Which has more protein?

    out of

12. The protein concentration difference on the two sides of the glomerular membranes causes a difference of osmotic pressure. This difference favors the movement of fluid from the filtrate back to

    the _____.

    blood in the capillaries

13. Does the effect of *capillary* osmotic pressure aid or oppose the hydrostatic driving force of filtration?

    blood (or capillaries)

14. The GFR (glomerular filtration rate) depends on blood pressure and on the concentration of

    _____ in the glomerular capillaries.

    opposes

15. The ultrafiltrate contains all the components of blood such as glucose, Na^+, K^+, Cl^-, urea, etc., except the cellular elements and large molecules,

    notably the _____.

    protein

16. Reabsorption and secretion of certain substances is the next process, after filtration, in the formation of urine by the functional unit of the kidney. This

    functional unit is called the _____.

    proteins

17. During the reabsorption process, the filtered substances pass either into or out of the surrounding
capillaries through the *tubule walls.* Most of the
filtered water is reabsorbed through the walls of

    the proximal _____. The final reabsorp-
tion of water occurs through the walls of the col-

    lecting _____.

18. About 99% of filtered water is reabsorbed over the
length of the nephron. Filtered glucose is usually
completely reabsorbed by the tubules and thus re-

    turned to the _____.

19. Other substances of the blood such as urea, uric
acid, SO_4^{-2}, K^+, and Mg^{+2} appear in the collecting
duct urine at a higher concentration than in the

    initial filtrate of the _____.

20. Thus we can see that if the renal tubules remove
more water than solutes from the filtrate, the *concentration* of these solutes in the tubular fluid will
have (increased/decreased) at the end of the
nephron.

21. Plasma clearance or simply *clearance* expresses the
ability of the kidney to remove various substances

    from the _____.

22. The ability of the kidneys to remove various substances from the blood or plasma is expressed as

    _____   _____.

23. Plasma clearance more accurately is a measure of
the volume of plasma which is cleared of a substance within a certain period of time. For example, if all of substance Z is removed from 1 liter of

    plasma in 1 hour, the clearance of Z is _____ liter

    per _____.

nephron

tubule
ducts

blood

glomerulus

increased

blood (plasma)

plasma clearance

153

24. Plasma clearance varies *directly* with the concentration of a substance in the *urine* and the *rate of urine flow* into the bladder. Thus when there is an *increase* in the concentration of a substance *in the urine* (and/or an increase in the rate of urine flow), plasma clearance can be expected to (increase/decrease).

1 hour

25. But plasma clearance varies *inversely* with the concentration of the substance *in the plasma.* Thus, if the concentration of the substance *in the plasma* is *high,* the plasma clearance would be (faster/slower) than if the concentration were low.

increase

26. Clearance of a substance is calculated by the following equation:

$$C = \frac{U \times V}{P}$$

slower

in which C = clearance (ml/min)
U = concentration of substance in the urine
V = rate of urine flow (ml/min)
P = concentration of substance in plasma

Example: the clearance of *urea* may be calculated from the following experimental data:

plasma concentration (P) = 26 mg% (mg per 100 ml solution)
urine concentration (U) = 1820 mg%
urine flow (V) = 1 ml/min

Solve for clearance (c).

27. Thus in this example, in one minute urea is cleared

from _____ ml of _____.

$$C = \frac{U \times V}{P}$$

$$\frac{1820 \times 1}{26} = 70 \text{ ml/min}$$

C = 70 ml/min

70, plasma

28. If a substance is filtered by the glomerulus, but is neither reabsorbed by nor secreted into the tubule,

then its _____, C, is a measure of the GFR.

NOTE: Inulin, a polysaccharide, is such a substance. It is neither secreted into nor reabsorbed from the tubular fluid. Thus inulin may be injected into the circulation; then its plasma and urine concentrations are measured, as is the urine flow rate. From this data, the clearance of inulin, which is equal to the GFR, is calculated. Clearance measurements provide useful information for diagnosing renal disease.

29. There are maximal rates of reabsorption or secretion of some substances through the tubule cells. This is called a tubular maximum, or Tm.

The maximal rate of reabsorption or secretion of a substance is called a _____ _____.

clearance

30. Glucose has a high Tm. So high, in fact that with normal blood glucose levels, glucose is completely

_____ through the tubule cells.

tubular maximum

31. However, when glucose has a high concentration in the plasma (as in untreated diabetes mellitus), its Tm may be exceeded.

When the Tm is exceeded, glucose is *not*

_____ reabsorbed and therefore appears in the _____.

reabsorbed

32. The kidney also regulates water and electrolyte concentrations of blood. It performs this regulatory function by controlling the levels of dissolved

substances in the _____.

completely
urine

33. Control is effected through changes in the rates at

which the kidney tubules _____ or secrete these substances.

blood (plasma)

155

34. Restating the fact, the rates of reabsorption and

_____ of various substances can be

changed. This affords a means of controlling the

_____ levels of these substances.

reabsorb

35. The reabsorption or the secretion of a substance
by the kidney tubule cells may be an *active* or a *passive* transport process. You'll recall that an *active*
transport process requires the expenditure of cellular energy; but a transport process which does not

require cellular energy is said to be _____.

secretion

blood

36. Which kind of reabsorptive process requires the
expenditure of cellular energy?

passive

37. Amino acids and glucose are among the more
important substances whose reabsorption requires
the expenditure of cellular energy. Thus we say

that these substances are _____
reabsorbed.

active

38. Active reabsorption of these substances takes place

in the proximal tubule of the _____.

actively

39. Na^+ (sodium ion) is actively reabsorbed from the
filtrate by both the *proximal* and the *distal*

_____ of the nephron as well as the
ascending limb of the loop of Henle.

nephron

40. Chloride ion (Cl^-) passively follows the active reabsorption of sodium ion (Na^+). This passive
movement of chloride ions (Cl^-) is in response to
the movement of sodium ion. This movement of
chloride is related to the (attraction/repulsion) of
unlike charges.

tubules

41. Water is passively _____ from the
tubule.

attraction

42. This passive reabsorption of water is in response to the osmotic pressure difference brought about by the _____ reabsorption of Na^+ and the _____ reabsorption of Cl^-.

reabsorbed (transported)

43. Thus, anything that interferes with the active reabsorption of Na^+ will also reduce the passive reabsorption of _____.

active
passive

44. If reabsorption of water is reduced, what effect will this have on the volume of urine that enters the bladder?

water

45. This increased urine formation is called *diuresis.* A diuretic, then, is a substance that causes

_____.

the volume is increased

46. Some diuretics (e.g., mercurial compounds) act by poisoning the metabolism, which supplies energy for the (active/passive) reabsorption of Na^+.

diuresis

47. Decreased Na^+ reabsorption then leads to a(n) (decreased/increased) water reabsorption and diuresis.

active

48. Another cause of _____ is injection of a substance into the blood stream which is poorly reabsorbed by the tubules from the glomerular filtrate.

decreased

49. Since little of this substance is reabsorbed from the tubule, its concentration in the tubular fluid will be (high/low).

diuresis

50. The reabsorption of water from the tubule is decreased because of the high solute concentration in the _____ fluid.

high

51. Less water reabsorption (increases/decreases) urine volume and is called _____.

tubular

157

52. Substances that cause less water to be reabsorbed from the tubules are called _____.

increases
diuresis

NOTE: *Examples of such "osmotic" diuretic substances include urea, sucrose, and mannitol. This same effect occurs when glucose rises to high levels in the blood as in diabetes mellitus. Above levels of about 250 mg%, glucose is poorly reabsorbed by the tubules and instead acts as an "osmotic" diuretic. "Diabetes" refers to the increased urine flow. Other substances such as caffeine, alcohol, and theophylline act as mild diuretics by increasing the glomerular filtration rate.*

53. The diagram below illustrates the mechanism of bicarbonate conservation by the kidney tubule:

diuretics

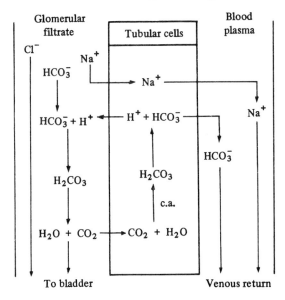

The inner side of the tubular cell (filtrate side) is relatively impermeable to the charged bicarbonate ion (HCO_3^-). Therefore little or none of this ion is

_____ by the tubular cells in the charged form.

54. However, the difficulty in transporting the charged Na^+ and H^+ is presumably overcome by the active

_____ processes for these ions.

reabsorbed

55. *Active* transport of Na^+ and H^+ requires the expenditure of cellular _____ .

transport

56. Refer to the diagram. You will see that between the filtrate and tubular cells Na^+ is exchanged for _____ .

energy

57. Na^+ (enters/leaves) the tubular cells and H^+ (leaves/enters) the cells to enter the _____ .

H^+

58. Then, the *secreted* H^+ combines with HCO_3^- in the filtrate to form _____ (check diagram), which breaks up into CO_2 and H_2O.

enters, leaves
filtrate

59. Now, we see that the uncharged CO_2 is readily absorbed from the filtrate into the _____ _____ .

H_2CO_3

60. And once inside the tubular cell, CO_2 combines with _____ to form H_2CO_3. (You'll recall that this reaction is facilitated by carbonic anhydrase. This enzyme is found in the *tubular cells*.)

tubular
cells

61. Next, the carbonic acid dissociates into H^+ and _____ .

H_2O

62. Finally, the H^+ is secreted into the _____ , and the HCO_3^- is *secreted* into the _____ _____ .

HCO_3^-

63. Thus, HCO_3^- reabsorption is dependent on the secretion of H^+ from the _____ _____ , which is dependent on the CO_2 supply in the _____ .

filtrate
blood
plasma

159

64. The level of CO_2 in the glomerular filtrate is related to the PCO_2 of the _____ from which
the filtrate was derived.

tubular cells
filtrate

65. As you may recall from your study of respiration,
an increased PCO_2 (as, e.g., from breath-holding)
causes an increase in blood acidity or a lowering of

blood _____.

blood (plasma)

66. Does a low pH indicate a high or low concentration
of H^+ in the blood?

pH

67. The renal response to increased PCO_2 of the blood
is to increase secretion of H^+. This increases the

amount of HCO_3^-, which is _____.

high

68. How do tubular H^+ secretion and HCO_3^- reabsorption affect blood pH?

reabsorbed

69. If you wish, you may review the effects of H^+
secretion and HCO_3^- reabsorption on blood pH
with respect to the following equation:

$$pH = pK + \log \frac{HCO_3^-}{H_2CO_3}$$

blood pH increases

70. When the excretion of bicarbonate is high, the
excretion of chloride is low. And, conversely, when
the excretion of bicarbonate is low the excretion
of chloride (increases/decreases).

71. Take another look at the previous diagram. Is Na^+
normally lost in the urine or retained by the body?

increases

72. Normally, Na^+ is (retained/lost) and H^+ is
(retained/lost).

retained

73. This is an exchange process: the tubule cells give

an H^+ to the filtrate in exchange for a _____,

which is _____ by the body.

(Na^+) retained
(H^+) lost

160

74. The handling of ammonia (NH_3) by the kidney is shown in the next diagram:

Na^+ retained

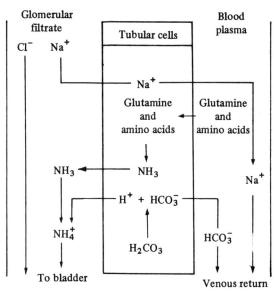

Ammonia (NH_3) is formed in the tubular cells from glutamine and amino acids. Then it is secreted into the _____ .

75. In the filtrate NH_3 combines with the secreted H^+ to form ammonium ion, _____ (the formula).

filtrate (tubule)

76. The _____ ion is then excreted along with Cl^-.

NH_4^+

77. Through a combination of events just described, the kidney regulates the pH of the _____ .

ammonium

78. All of the filtered HCO_3^- is recovered, and H^+ secretion is increased when the blood pH becomes low (acidosis). Thus, the increased secretion of H^+ will (raise/lower) blood pH toward a normal value of 7.4.

blood

79. Most of the *water* of the ultrafiltrate is reabsorbed from the proximal renal tubule. However, water reabsorption also occurs from the _____ tubules and the _____ ducts.

80. Water reabsorption from these areas is under the control of the antidiuretic hormone (ADH) from the posterior pituitary gland. Release of the anti_____hormone is regulated by impulses from *osmoreceptor* cells near the pituitary and from blood volume receptors in the chest.

81. This hormone release system is diagrammed below:

When you drink a large amount of water that is not needed by the body you (increase/decrease) the volume of body water and (increase/decrease) the concentration of plasma electrolytes.

82. The *blood volume receptors* in the chest respond to the increased blood _____, and the *osmotic receptors* respond to the decreased _____ of electrolytes.

83. Both factors *inhibit* the release of the pituitary hormone known as _____.

162

84. Thus, the decreased ADH level reduces the reabsorption of water by the distal renal _____
and the _____ _____.

ADH

85. Since *less* water is reabsorbed by the tubules, the
volume of water that passes into the ureters and
bladder is (smaller/greater).

tubules
collecting ducts

86. Most of the Na$^+$ in the filtrate is reabsorbed by the
proximal _____.

greater

87. Some Na$^+$ is also reabsorbed by the distal tubule.
But, here Na$^+$ reabsorption is stimulated by
aldosterone from the *adrenal cortex*.

tubule

NOTE: Abnormal constituents that may appear in urine include protein (indicative of kidney disease), glucose (diabetes mellitus), hemoglobin (red cell destruction), bile (jaundice), and certain amino acids (indicative of metabolic problems).

88. Here's a brief review before you complete this section. The kidney is made up of functional units
called _____.

89. The rate at which filtration occurs in the nephron
is called the _____ _____ _____.

nephrons

90. Clearance is calculated from urine concentration,
_____ flow rate, and _____
_____.

GFR or glomerular
filtration rate

91. By the tubular cells, hydrogen ion is exchanged for
_____ ion.

urine, plasma
concentration

92. Chloride excretion is inversely proportional to
_____ ion secretion.

sodium

163

93. Water reabsorption from the collecting ducts and distal tubules is regulated by the hormone

_____ .

bicarbonate

94. Blood *p*H is regulated by the functions of both the _____ (organ) and the _____ (organ).

ADH

lungs, kidneys

This completes your study of Renal Physiology in Section VI. After a short break, continue with Section VII, Digestion.

DIGESTION

Digestion is the preparation of food for absorption into the body. After entering the mouth, food is chewed, mixed with saliva, and formed into a bolus or ball which is pushed into the pharynx by the swallowing reflex. This reflex is initiated voluntarily but the remainder of the swallowing reflex is involuntary. The bolus is prevented from entering the larynx and trachea by the epiglottis and by the temporary cessation of breathing. The bolus enters the esophagus and is carried to the stomach by peristaltic (wave-like) action.

1. As the food passes along the *digestive* tract it is acted upon by enzymes which break down part of the food preparatory to absorption. The food that is not *digested* (broken down) passes through

   the digestive tract and is _____ in the feces.

2. Foods are classified into three main classes: *carbohydrates, proteins,* and *fats.* Sugars and starches belong to the class of foods known as _____.

   excreted (discharged)

3. *Glucose* is the usual end product of the *digestion*

   of _____.

   carbohydrates

4. *Glucose* is the usual end product of carbohydrate

   _____.

   carbohydrates

165

5. Thus, the most prevalent carbohydrate form found in the blood is ——————.

6. *Proteins* are complex molecules composed of *amino acids.* The end products of protein digestion are a variety of —————— acids.

7. Fats are composed of *fatty acids* and *glycerol.* A fat, which is composed of *three* fatty acids (the same or different), connected to *one* glycerol molecule, is termed a (di-/triglyceride).

8. The skeletal structure of a triglyceride is given below.

$$
\begin{array}{l}
H \\
HC - O - X_1 \\
| \\
HC - O - X_2 \\
| \\
HC - O - X_3 \\
H
\end{array}
$$

Triglyceride

$$X_1, X_2, X_3 = \text{fatty acids}$$

Some fat is absorbed as triglyceride, some is absorbed with one fatty acid split off (diglyceride), some with two fatty acids split offs (mono-/diglyceride), and some as glycerol and free fatty

——————.

9. The secretion of saliva in the mouth is controlled by *parasympathetic* activity.

   The presence of *food* in the mouth leads to an increase in saliva secretion because its presence activates the —————————— system.

10. What process is facilitated by the lubricating action of saliva?

166

11. But saliva has another function. It contains the
enzyme, salivary amylase, which begins the break-

ing down or _____ of starch.

swallowing

12. One function of the stomach is to store food
awaiting passage into the duodenum. The large
amount of food swallowed at a meal enters the

esophagus and moves into the _____.
Then by peristalsis, the food slowly passes through

the remainder of the _____ tract.

digesting

13. The gastric juices are mixed with the food by con-

tractions of the _____. Hydrochloric
acid (HCl) and a protein-splitting enzyme, *pepsin,*
are part of the _____ juice.

stomach
digestive

14. An *enzyme* that breaks proteins into smaller

molecules is _____.

stomach
gastric

15. The *p*H of the stomach contents is about 2, which
is highly acidic. The presence of food in the *mouth*
initiates the secretion of gastric juice in the

_____.

pepsin

16. The vagus nerve carries the impulse to the secre-

tory cells of the _____ wall.

stomach

17. The continued secretion of *gastric* _____
depends on the release of the hormone *gastrin* by
cells in the stomach and duodenum.

stomach

18. *Gastrin,* released into the blood stream, stimulates
the secretory cells of the stomach and duodenum

to continue the secretion of _____

_____.

juice

19. The hormone that makes possible the continued

    release of gastric juice is _____.

20. When fat is present in the stomach contents, a sec-
    ond hormone is released by the stomach and
    duodenum into the circulation. This enzyme is
    called *enterogastrone*.

    The hormone released by the stomach and duode-
    num due to the presence of fat, which inhibits the

    activity of the stomach, is_____.

21. Thus, the hormone that inhibits the activity of the

    stomach is _____.

22. Since this hormone inhibits the stomach activity,
    it delays the emptying of the stomach contents
    into the next portion of the digestive tract, which

    is the _____.

23. The gastric glands also produce a substance called

    the *intrinsic factor*. This _____ factor
    facilitates the absorption of vitamin B_{12}.

24. *Bile* from the *liver* and *pancreatic juice* from the

    _____ enter the duodenum via the
    common bile duct.

    The common bile duct delivers, to the duodenum,

    the _____ (from the liver) and _____
    juice (from the pancreas).

25. Food in the duodenum initiates the release of two
    hormones, *secretin* and *pancreozymin,* by the
    duodenal cells. Then, the two hormones, secretin

    and _____ stimulate the release of
    the *pancreatic* juice into duodenum.

26. The hormones that stimulate the secretion of pancreatic juice are _____ and

_____ .

pancreozymin

27. In addition, stimulation of the vagus _____ induces a small amount of pancreatic secretion.

secretin
pancreozymin

28. Pancreatic juice contains *enzymes* that break down all three classes of foods—that is, proteins, lipids

(fats), and _____ .

nerves

29. Pancreatic juice also contains sodium bicarbonate, which neutralizes the HCl delivered to the duodenum along with food from the _____ .

carbohydrates

30. A compound that neutralizes the HCl carried to the duodenum along with food from the stomach

is _____ bicarbonate.

stomach

31. The *gall bladder* stores the bile, which is continu-

ously produced by the _____ .

sodium

32. When fat-rich food enters the duodenum, the hormone *cholecystokinin* is released into the circulation. Cholecystokinin causes the gall bladder to contract and discharge its contents, that is, dis-

charge _____ into the duodenum via the common bile duct.

liver

33. The principal active ingredients of bile are the *bile salts,* primarily sodium glycocholate and sodium taurocholate.

The digestion of fat is aided by these bile _____ .

bile

34. First, the bile salts *emulsify* the _____ . Then, in combination with the fat-splitting enzymes

(lipases), they permit the _____ to be absorbed.

salts

169

35. The very small droplets of fat arising from the emulsifying action of the _____ _____ are absorbed into the lymphatic system.

fat
fat(s)

36. Fat droplets pass through the intestinal lacteals into the *lymphatic system.*

This absorbed fat passes through the thoracic duct of the _____ system and then into the left subclavian *vein.*

bile salts

37. Fat is then transported to all parts of the body via the circulation of _____.

lymphatic

38. Some fat, which has been broken down further into diglycerides and _____, is absorbed into the bloodstream directly from the intestine. Fat is also absorbed as

_____ (third type).

blood

39. Some additional enzymes are secreted by the small intestine itself and aid in the process of

_____.

monoglycerides
triglyceride

40. The rate at which food is propelled through the small _____ is regulated by the sympathetic and parasympathetic _____ system.

digestion

41. Stimulation of the *sympathetic* system *reduces* intestinal peristalsis. On the other hand, activity of the parasympathetic system (increases/decreases) the peristaltic movement of food along the small intestine.

intestine
nervous

42. Peristaltic movement of food *decreases* with

stimulation of the _____ system,
whereas activity of the *parasympathetic* nervous

system _____ intestinal peristalsis.

43. The absorption of digested food occurs primarily

in the small _____.

44. Undigested, unabsorbed food passes from the small

intestine into the _____ intestine.

45. A reflex initiated by the entry of food into the
stomach brings about peristalsis of the large

_____.

46. Thus, when additional food enters the stomach,

_____ increases in the large intestine.

47. The food residue is pushed along the large intestine

by the process of _____ and is
discharged from the body as *feces.*

48. *Feces* consist of undigested food (mainly cellu-
lose), a large amount of bacteria (normally present
and multiplying in the intestine), various insoluble
or poorly absorbed substances, cellular fragments,
and derivatives of bile.

The amount of bile lost in the feces is small since
most of it is reabsorbed from the intestine and re-

turned via the circulation to the _____ for
resecretion.

49. The water content of feces depends in part on the

osmotic _____ differences occurring
across the gut (intestinal) wall.

increases

sympathetic
increases

intestine

large

intestine

peristalsis

peristalsis

liver

50. The gut concentration of unabsorbed salts affects

the _____ pressure difference across the
gut wall.

pressure

51. Magnesium sulfate is an example of a poorly ab-

sorbed _____.

osmotic

52. A salt that retains water in the intestine and thus

acts as a laxative is magnesium _____.

salt

53. The expulsion of feces, or *defecation,* in the adult
is under voluntary control via action of the puden-
dal nerve on the external anal sphincter. Contract-
ing the diaphragm and the abdominal muscles
increases abdominal pressure and thus may aid

_____ (the expulsion of feces).

sulfate

54. In summary, digestion prepares food for absorption

by the _____ intestine. Digestive _____
are reflexly secreted into the digestive tract. These
reflex secretions are brought about by the

_____ system and by the release of certain

_____ into the circulation in response to
the presence of food in the digestive tract. The
movement of food through the tract occurs by

_____. Undigested or unabsorbed

food is expelled as _____.

defecation

small, enzymes
nervous
hormones
peristalsis
feces

This completes a very short section on Digestion. Go on to Section VIII, Endo-
crinology.

SECTION VIII

ENDOCRINOLOGY

The glands of the body are of two types, the exocrines and the endocrines. The exocrine glands secrete externally. Examples of exocrine glands are the sweat glands, the mammary glands, and the glands of the stomach and intestine. These glands pass their secretions through ducts either to the external surface of the body or to the digestive tract.

The endocrine glands are ductless. Their secretions are passed directly into the bloodstream and are transmitted via the circulation to modify the activity of various organs and tissues of the body. The endocrine glands provide an additional means of control for the body. The nervous system provides rapid control; the endocrine system exerts its control more slowly.

✗ 1. Endocrine glands secrete directly into the

_____ .

2. Endocrine glands secrete directly into the blood   bloodstream

stream; exocrine glands secrete _____ .

✗ 3. Hormones are the secretions of endocrine glands.   externally

Hormones are secreted _____ into the
bloodstream.   directly

*NOTE: The endocrine glands of the body and the hormones they secrete are given
in the following table:*

ENDOCRINE GLANDS AND HORMONES

Gland	Hormone(s)*

Pituitary (anterior)	Growth hormone (GH, STH)
	Thyrotrophic hormone (TSH)
	Adrenocorticotrophic hormone (ACTH)
	Gonadotrophic hormones
	  (a) Follicle stimulating hormone (FSH)
	  (b) Luteinizing hormone (prolactin, LH)
	  (c) Luteotrophic hormone (LTH)

Pituitary (posterior)	Antidiuretic hormones (vasopressin, ADH) Oxytocin
Thyroid	Thyroxin (T-4)
Parathyroid	Parathyroid hormones (PTH)
Adrenal (medulla)	Epinephrine Norepinephrine
Adrenal (cortex)	Adrenal steroids
Pancreas (islets)	Insulin Glucagon
Gonads (male)	Testosterone
(female)	Estrogen Progesterone
Placenta	Gonadotrophins Progesterone

*Synonyms for the hormones are given in parentheses.

4. The anatomical description of the endocrine glands should be reviewed at this point. In the next section we shall discuss the functions of these glands.

✗ 5. The pituitary gland (hypophysis) consists of anterior and _____ portions.

6. The anterior portion of the pituitary gland secretes growth hormone and the following trophic hormones: thyrotrophic hormone, adrenocorticotrophic hormone, and the gonadotrophic hormones. The entire pituitary gland is called the

_____.

posterior

7. A *trophic* hormone is one that acts on another endocrine gland causing it to secrete its

_____.

hypophysis

8. A hormone that acts upon another endocrine gland causing it to secrete is a _____ hormone.

hormone(s)

9. For example, adrenocorticotrophic hormone (ACTH) causes the adrenal cortex to release certain of its steroid _____.

trophic

10. What gland produces ACTH?

hormones

11. Although the trophic hormones act on specific endocrine _____ (target glands) they may also exert actions at other sites in the body.

anterior pituitary

12. The *specific* glands acted on by trophic hormones are called _____ glands.

glands

13. For example, thyrotrophic hormone [thyroid stimulating hormone (TSH)] controls the activity of the _____ gland.

target

14. Therefore, overproduction of TSH leads to overactivity of the _____ _____.

thyroid

15. If the anterior pituitary were surgically removed, would the thyroid glands secrete more or less thyroxin?

thyroid gland

175

16. Adrenocorticotrophic hormone (ACTH) controls the release of certain steroids from the cortex of the _____ gland.

less, due to lack of stimulus from TSH

17. That is, release of *steroid* hormones from the adrenal cortex increases when ACTH release is (increased/decreased).

adrenal

18. Thus, decreased ACTH in the circulation leads to a (increase/decrease) in adrenal steroid release from the cortex.

increased

19. The *gonadotrophic* hormones consist of follicle stimulating hormone (FSH), luteinizing hormone (LH), and luteotrophic hormone (LTH). The endocrine and reproductive activity of the ovaries and the testes are controlled by the gonadotrophic

_____.

decrease

20. Or we say that the gonadotrophic hormones control the endocrine and reproductive activity of the

_____ and _____.

hormones

21. The posterior portion of the _____ secretes antidiuretic hormone (ADH) and oxytocin.

ovaries, testes

22. Thus, ADH regulates the reabsorption of water from the distal tubules and collecting ducts of the kidney. In this way ADH from the posterior

_____ regulates the volume of urine

passing from the _____ to the bladder.

pituitary
(hypophysis)

23. A deficiency of ADH permits an increased loss of water in the urine by *decreasing* tubular water reabsorption. Thus, a deficiency of ADH leads to diabetes insipidus in which (large/small) volumes of dilute urine are passed.

pituitary
kidneys

24. Can you think of a treatment for diabetes insipidus?

large

25. Although large injected doses of ADH cause vasoconstriction and a rise in blood pressure, the nor-

administer ADH

mal amounts secreted by the posterior _____
show little of this *vasopressor* activity.

26. Consequently *ADH* is a more appropriate term

pituitary

than vasopressin for this _____. (Refer
to the endocrine and hormone table following
Frame 3.)

27. Oxytocin has a chemical structure very similar to
that of ADH. Oxytocin causes contraction of the
pregnant uterus and is often used to induce the
onset of labor and to enhance uterine contractions
during labor. *Milk ejection* by the mammary
glands following childbirth is another effect of
oxytocin.

hormone

The posterior pituitary releases two hormones,

_____ and _____, but they are
manufactured in the *hypothalamus* of the brain.

28. ADH and oxytocin are released from the

ADH, oxytocin

_____ _____, but are

manufactured in the _____.

*NOTE: ADH and oxytocin are manufactured in the hypothalamus and transported
to the posterior pituitary through the* nerves *connecting the hypothalamus and
posterior pituitary—the hypothalamo-hypophyseal tracts. Some storage of these
hormones occurs prior to their release. Release is effected by nervous stimuli to
the posterior pituitary.*

29. Growth hormone (somatotrophic hormone—STH)
is released by another portion of the hypophysis

posterior pituitary
hypothalamus

known as the _____ _____.

30. STH is called the _____ hormone.   anterior pituitary

31. Although one's size is determined primarily by   growth
    inherited factors, an additional factor during the

    growth period is the amount of circulating _____.

32. Thus, underproduction of this hormone (STH)   STH

    during the growth years leads to retarded _____
    and dwarfism.

33. Name a possible cause of gigantism.   growth

34. Overproduction of STH later in life leads to a re-   overproduction of STH
    newed growth of the bones of the hands, feet and
    head but not of the long bones of the limbs which
    have lost the power to grow. *Acromegaly* is the
    term used to describe the increase in size of hands,

    feet, and head due to overproduction of _____.

35. The trophic hormones of the anterior _____   STH
    are released in response to lowered levels of hor-
    mones produced by the target glands.

36. Accordingly, an *increased* production of hormone   pituitary
    by the target gland leads to a(n) (increased/de-
    creased) production of the specific trophic hor-
    mone involved.

37. *Negative feedback* is the term that describes this   decreased
    reciprocal control between the trophic

    _____ from the _____ and

    the hormone produced by the _____
    gland.

38. For example, when a thermostat turns on a furnace, heat is sent throughout the house. Some of
this heat reaches the thermostat, which then turns
off the furnace. Thus, the relation between a furnace and its controlling thermostat is a form of

negative _____.

hormone, pituitary
target

39. An endocrine example of negative feedback is the
relation between the thyroid gland and the

_____ gland.

feedback

40. Let's take a closer look at an endocrine example
of negative feedback. The thyroid gland is induced
to secrete *thyroxin* by TSH from the anterior lobe

of the _____.

pituitary

41. As the level of thyroxin in the blood *increases,* the
secretion of TSH (increases/decreases).

pituitary

Hypothalamus

Negative feedback

*NOTE: Negative feedback is also evident in the control of the release of certain
adrenal steroids and gonadal steroids. The* posterior *lobe hormones are released in
response to stimuli from the nervous system.*

42. Now let's discuss the thyroid gland and the hormone
it produces—thyroxin.

decreases

43. The thyroid hormone, or _____, is made from the amino acid *tyrosine* and *iodine,* which the thyroid concentrates from the blood.

Thyroxin is made from tyrosine and _____ in the thyroid gland.

44. After thyroxin is synthesized from _____

and _____, it is combined with a protein and stored in a form called *thyroglobulin.*

45. Before release into the circulation, a plasma en-

zyme splits the stored _____ into *thyroxin* and the *protein* to which it was bound.

46. Thyroxin stimulates metabolism in all body tissues. Therefore, what is its effect on oxygen consumption and heat production by the body tissues?

47. The *basal metabolic rate* (BMR) is the body's energy requirement at rest.

The body's basic energy requirement at rest is the

_____ _____ _____.

48. The normal level of circulating thyroxin maintains

a basal metabolic rate (abbr. _____) which for males is about 40 calories per square meter of body surface per hour.

49. The normal basal _____rate for females is about 37 cal/m^2/hr.

50. An increased thyroxin output (increases/ decreases) the BMR; the BMR decreases when the

output of _____ decreases.

51. Basal energy requirements depend on a person's size and are most closely related to the person's body surface area. Consequently, for comparison between persons, the basal _____ _____ is expressed in terms of body surface area or square _____ (m^2).

increases
thyroxin

52. Thus, BMR is expressed as $cal/m^2/hr$, that is, the energy utilized per _____ meter per _____.

metabolic
rate
meters

53. $Cal/m^2/hr$ is an expression of _____.

square
hour

54. *Goiter* (or increase in size) may be associated with either overactivity or underactivity of the thyroid _____.

BMR

55. An increase in the size of the thyroid gland is called a _____.

gland

56. Overactivity of the thyroid gland is called *hyper-thyroidism* or, if the condition is more serious, *thyrotoxicosis*. Thyrotoxicosis may result from a tumor in the thyroid or from an excess of TSH from the anterior _____ gland.

goiter

57. One symptom of thyrotoxicosis is a BMR up to 50% above normal. Nervousness, tremors, increased excitability of heart muscle, and protrusion of the eyeballs (exophthalmos) are other symptoms that may indicate a condition of _____.

pituitary

58. Surgical removal of part of the thyroid is a possible treatment for (hypo-/hyperthyroidism).

thyrotoxicosis

59. Another treatment is to destroy part of the gland by a radioactive element. What element, because of its concentration by the thyroid, is a logical choice for an attack on the thyroid?

hyperthyroidism

60. In addition, antithyroid agents such as *thiouracil* or *thiocyanate* may be used. These substances reduce the thyroid's synthesis of its hormone,

_____.

radioactive iodine

61. Underactivity of the thyroid gland is called *hypothyroidism*. *Cretins* are individuals who are born with an underactive thyroid. They are small, mentally retarded, and usually have a large protruding tongue. This condition is also known as (hypo-/ hyperthyroidism).

thyroxin

62. Suggest a possible treatment for such a child.

hypothyroidism

63. A thyroid deficiency later in life leads to myxedema. Is myxedema characterized by a high or low BMR?

administer thyroxin or TSH

64. Thus, later in life, hypothyroidism which manifests itself in slow speech and movement and an increase in weight is characteristic of _____.

low

65. Myxedema may be treated by administration of

_____.

myxedema

66. Hypothyroidism, associated with goiter, may be due to a dietary deficiency of what element?

thyroxin (TSH)

67. Consequently what element is often added to table salt to prevent this deficiency?

iodine

68. The parathyroid glands, located on the thyroid gland, secrete the parathyroid _____.

iodine

69. Parathormone (PTH), as the parathyroid hormone is sometimes called, is a protein and is inactive when taken by mouth.

The hormone secreted by the parathyroid gland is

_____ (PTH).

70. Underactivity of the parathyroid gland leads to a *decreased* loss of phosphate through the kidneys. Thus the level of phosphate in the blood (increases/ decreases).

71. Underactivity of the parathyroid gland leads to an

increased level in the blood of _____.

72. The altered phosphate level is accompanied by a lowered blood calcium level (hypocalcemia). If the blood calcium level drops a sufficient amount, muscle *tetany* occurs. In tetany there is an increased excitability of nerves and neuromuscular junctions leading to muscle spasm, especially of the hands and feet (carpopedal spasm).

This blood calcium level is related to the rate of calcium absorption from the intestine and to the rate of calcium excretion through the

_____.

73. Blood calcium level is also related to the rate at

which _____ is *deposited* in or *resorbed* from bone.

74. Study the following diagram, which outlines the factors affecting blood calcium level:

An excess of parathormone increases *resorption* of *bone.* How does this affect the calcium level in the blood?

183

75. Cyst formation in the bone and a tendency toward spontaneous fractures usually result from resorption of calcium from _____.

calcium level is increased

76. The intestinal absorption of calcium is facilitated by *vitamin D.*

Name an excellent dietary source of calcium and also the vitamin which is often added to it.

bone

77. Decreased calcium levels due to impaired absorption from the intestine is a cause of rickets in children. What vitamin might be prescribed in the treatment of rickets?

milk, vitamin D

78. Now let's take a closer look at the endocrine glands called the adrenals. These glands consist of two parts: the central part or *medulla* and the outer part or *cortex.* The medulla is the (central/outer) part of the adrenal, and is stimulated by *preganglionic sympathetic nerves* to secrete *epinephrine* and *norepinephrine.*

vitamin D

79. The adrenal medulla is stimulated by preganglionic _____ nerves to secrete *epinephrine* and nor _____.

central

80. The adrenal medulla is activated by the conditions of cold, low blood sugar, fear, low blood pressure, anger, and asphyxia.

When the adrenal medulla is activated it secretes _____ and _____.

sympathetic
norepinephrine

81. Epinephrine and norepinephrine are known as *catecholamines.* Some general actions of the catecholamines are given in the next table:

epinephrine
norepinephrine

184

EFFECTS OF EPINEPHRINE AND NOREPINEPHRINE

Function	Effect	
	Epinephrine	Norepinephrine
Peripheral resistance	decreased	increased
Systolic blood pressure	increased	increased
Heart rate	increased	—
Coronary vessels	dilated	dilated
Bronchial muscles	inhibition	inhibition
Blood sugar	increased	increased
Mental state	anxiety	—
Skeletal muscle blood flow	increased	—
Brain blood flow	increased	—
Kidney blood flow	decreased	slight decrease

82. Catecholamines act on two types of receptor sites in the circulatory system, designated α (alpha) receptors and β (beta) _____.

83. The α-_____ are associated with the contraction of smooth _____ found in the arterioles, whereas the β-receptors are associated with the *inhibition* or *relaxation* of smooth muscle in the _____.

    receptors

84. The α-receptors are associated with the *contraction* of arteriolar smooth muscle, whereas β-receptors are associated with the _____ or _____ of this smooth muscle.

    receptors
    muscle
    arterioles

85. The α-receptors are associated with the _____ of arteriolar smooth muscle.

    inhibition
    relaxation

86. The receptors associated with inhibition of smooth muscle are ____- receptors.

    contraction

NOTE: In addition, these receptors are associated with an increase in the force of contraction of the heart and an increase in heart rate.

185

87. The adrenal cortex is not under direct control of the nervous system. Instead it is partly under the hormonal control of the anterior _____ gland.

88. Name the pituitary trophic hormone that controls the adrenal cortex.

89. The adrenal cortex produces three classes of steroid hormones:
    (a) glucocorticoids
    (b) mineralocorticoids
    (c) sex steroids

    Cortisol (hydrocortisone) is the primary *glucocorticoid* produced by the _____ _____.

90. The *glucocorticoids* regulate the metabolism of carbohydrates, proteins, and fats. Thus, the increased breakdown of tissue protein to *amino acids* is the result of (increased/decreased) secretion of

    _____.

91. Increased secretion of glucocorticoids leads to an increased breakdown of tissue protein to

    _____ _____.

92. These *amino acids* are converted to *glycogen* and blood glucose in the liver. Thus, in the liver, amino acids are converted to _____ and blood

    _____ .

93. In addition, fat is mobilized from its storage depots and converted in part to *ketone* bodies (β-hydroxy-butyrate, acetoacetate, and acetone). Thus, increased secretion of glucocorticoids from the adrenal cortex can lead to a(n) (increase/decrease) of these ketone bodies—a condition called *ketosis.*

β

pituitary

ACTH

adrenal cortex

increased
glucocorticoids

amino acids

glycogen
glucose

94. *Diabetes mellitus* is sometimes associated with hypersecretion of the glucocorticoids. Hypersecretion of the glucocorticoids leads to an increase in blood sugar levels. A high blood sugar level together with ketosis is a type of _____ mellitus.

increase

95. What type of diabetes results from a deficiency of ADH from the anterior pituitary?

diabetes

96. Diabetes mellitus is usually associated with a lack of insulin from the pancreas, although it may be the result of hypersecretion of the adrenal

_____ (Cushing's disease).

diabetes insipidus

97. Glucocorticoids reduce the swelling associated with a minor injury such as a splinter or insect bite.

Thus, the hormones which act to inhibit the walling-off process that normally occurs to isolate an injury are the _____.

cortex

98. Aldosterone and deoxycorticosterone (DOC) are the most prominent mineralocorticoids produced

by the _____ _____.

glucocorticoids

99. As you might expect, sodium and potassium levels of the blood are regulated by the

_____.

adrenal cortex

100. However, aldosterone and DOC act principally to regulate the *sodium ion.* Both hormones stimulate the reabsorption of sodium from the kidney tubule

and decrease the _____ ion concentration of sweat.

mineralocorticoids

101. The excretion of potassium by the kidneys is *increased* under the influence of the hormones known

as _____.

sodium

102. Thus, the mineralocorticoids influence the kidneys to reabsorb _____ and to increase the excretion of _____.

mineralocorticoids

103. What *pituitary* hormone stimulates the adrenal cortex?

Mineralocorticoid secretion from the _____

_____ is an exception—it is not under the direct control of _____.

sodium
potassium

104. The secretion of mineralocorticoids is related to the osmotic pressure of the blood which is in turn a function of the concentrations of the ions of

_____ and _____.

adrenal
cortex
ACTH

105. Underactivity of the _____ cortex is called *Addison's disease* and if untreated may prove fatal.

sodium
potassium

106. Low blood pressure, muscle weakness, skin pigmentation, and an excessive loss of sodium chloride in the urine are characteristics of _____ disease, resulting from adrenocortical

_____ activity.

adrenal

107. In addition to the glucocorticoids and mineralocorticoids, *sex hormones* are also produced by the

_____ _____.

Addison's
*under*activity

108. However, production of sex hormones in the adrenals is unimportant relative to the larger quantities of sex hormones (steroids) produced by the

_____.

adrenal cortex

109. On the other hand, certain tumors of the adrenal cortex may lead to an increased production of the

_____ hormones.

gonads

188

110. The result may be precocious puberty in children, virilism in adult females, or feminization in adult

_____.

sex

111. Two hormones are associated with the *islet cells* of the pancreas. *Insulin* is produced in the β-cells and *glucagon* in the α-cells.

Glucagon is produced in the α-cells whereas insulin is produced in the _____-cells.

males

112. Which islet-cell type failure would result in diabetes mellitus?

β

113. A deficiency of circulating insulin results in high blood sugar, fatigue, loss of weight, and ketosis. Name the disease implied by these symptoms.

β-cells (insulin)

114. With insufficient circulating insulin, fat is not metabolized through the normal pathways and as a consequence *ketone bodies* are formed. Thus, a decrease in blood *p*H (acidosis), which may produce coma, may result from the accumulation in

the blood of these _____ bodies.

diabetes mellitus

115. What hormone is given to diabetics, restoring their ability to utilize carbohydrates?

ketone

116. An excess of insulin leads to a low blood sugar, sweating, and ultimately to coma due to the low

blood level of _____.

insulin

117. Glucagon from the α-cells of the pancreatic islets facilitates the conversion of liver glycogen to blood glucose. Does glucagon raise or lower the blood sugar level?

sugar (glucose)

118. Let's go on to the sex hormones (sex steroids) which are produced by the ovaries and the testes. You may recall that small amounts of sex hormones are also produced by the _____

_____.

raises it

119. The ovaries produce *estrogens* and *progestogens,*

which are two types of ——————— ———————.

adrenal
cortex

120. *Estrogens* and *progestogens* are made primarily by
what glands?

sex hormones

The hormonal relations among the ovary, uterus,
and pituitary are summarized in the figure below.
Refer to this figure to help you respond to any of
the next few frames covering our discussion of sex
hormones:

ovaries

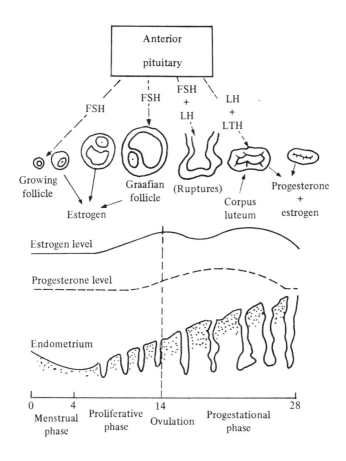

190

121. The pituitary gonadotrophins, FSH, LH, and, to
some extent, LTH, act on the ovaries to regulate

the production of _____ and

_____.

122. One function of the ovaries is the production of   estrogens
eggs or ova. After puberty, in a cyclic fashion with   progestogens
an average cycle length of about 28 days, the

ovaries produce and release _____.

123. The *menstrual cycle* is the term used to describe   ova (eggs)
the associated changes in the uterus, and this

cyclic release of _____ by the _____.

124. Thus, the interplay of the hormones from the   ova (eggs), ovaries
ovaries and the gonadotrophins from the pituitary

regulate the _____ cycle.

125. During the menstrual _____ the lining (endo-   menstrual
metrium) of the uterus undergoes cyclic changes

due to the ovarian _____. (see
Frame 120)

126. The menstrual cycle is divided into four phases: cycle
the *menstrual* phase, the *proliferative* phase, the   hormones

ovulatory _____, and the *progestational*

_____.

127. The beginning of the menstrual phase (called   phase
day 1) continues for 4 to 5 days. *Menstruation* is   phase
the loss of blood which characterizes this

_____ phase.

128. The bleeding of the menstrual phase results from a   menstrual
regression and surface disintegration of the endo-

metrium of the _____.

129. The *proliferative* phase is governed by the *estrogens* and lasts from the end of menstrual disintegration of the endometrium to the release of another

_____ by an ovary. (refer to Frame 120)

uterus

130. Normally an ovum is released by only one ovary during each _____ *cycle.*

ovum (egg)

131. The proliferative phase is controlled by the hormones called _____.

menstrual

132. The first phase of the menstrual cycle is called the _____ phase. This phase is followed by the _____ phase.

estrogens

133. The *proliferative* phase lasts about 10 days. The level of estrogen in the blood rises during this phase. In response to the increased estrogen levels, the *endometrium* of the uterus undergoes changes to prepare it for the possible arrival of a fertilized

_____.

menstrual
proliferative

134. Thus, the proliferative phase is characterized by a thickening and vascularization of the uterine

_____. (see illustration, Frame 120)

ovum (egg)

135. The release of an egg is called *ovulation.* Although there is a great deal of variation of this timing among different women, ovulation occurs about

the 14th day of the menstrual _____.

endometrium

136. The *ovulatory* phase is followed by the *progestational* _____, which lasts until the next menstrual phase.

cycle

137. After the proliferative phase comes _____ and then the _____ phase.

phase

138. During the *progestational* phase the uterine

_____ differentiates into a highly

vascular and glandular tissue.

ovulation

progestational

139. During the progestational phase preparation pro-
gresses for the implantation of a fertilized

_____.

endometrium

*NOTE: The fertilized ovum will have already undergone several divisions before
reaching the uterine endometrium and consequent implantation.*

140. The progestational phase occurs under the influ-

ence of both the estrogens and the _____.

ovum

141. If fertilization of an ovum and its implantation do
not occur during the progestational phase, the

endometrium of the _____ begins to dis-

integrate and the next _____ period
begins.

progestogens

142. Menstrual cycles in humans continue for about 35
years, after which time ovulation and the

_____ cycles cease.

uterus

menstrual

143. *Menopause* is the term used to indicate cessation

of ovulation and the _____ _____.

menstrual

144. The development of an ovum and the growth of
the endometrium during the proliferative phase
are stimulated by FSH from the anterior

_____.

menstrual

cycle

145. The ovum develops in a small sac in the _____
called a Graafian follicle.

pituitary

146. At *ovulation,* the Graafian _____
ruptures, normally releasing the egg.

ovary

193

147. The ovum then moves along the Fallopian tube to the uterus. Following this release of an egg, called

_____, the influence of the luteinizing hormone (LH) changes the ruptured Graafian

_____ into a corpus luteum.

follicle

148. LTH from the pituitary then stimulates the corpus luteum to produce the other type of ovarian hormone called _____.

ovulation
follicle

149. As the corpus luteum degenerates toward the end of the progestational phase, the level of the hormone _____ falls. (refer to Frame 120)

progesterone

150. The falling progesterone level leads to the shedding of the *endometrium* of the uterus and thus the onset of _____.

progesterone

151. The progestational phase is maintained if the _____ is fertilized and implants in the _____ of the uterus.

menstruation

152. The menstrual cycles cease during pregnancy. Thus, until after birth the ovaries normally do not release any _____.

ovum
endometrium

153. The increased levels of progestogens maintain the smooth muscle of the uterus in a "quiet" state of reduced contractility. The developing *embryo* forms two membranes to surround it, the *chorion* and the *amnion*.

One of the two membranes enveloping the embryo is the *chorion* and the other is the _____.

ova

154. A part of the chorion develops into the *placenta,* which provides nourishment for and removes wastes from the growing _____.

amnion

194

155. The placenta also produces estrogens, progestogens, and gonadotrophic hormones similar to LH. Thus, the placenta also acts as an endocrine _____.

embryo

156. The gonadotrophic _____ produced by the placenta are called *chorionic* gonadotrophins.

gland

157. During early pregnancy, high levels of *chorionic* _____ appear in the maternal urine.

hormones

158. Thus, to ascertain the condition of pregnancy, a urine test can be made to determine the presence of these _____ gonadotrophins.

gonadotrophins

159. Childbirth (parturition) is brought about by the intermittent contractions of the uterine wall. The mature fetus is expelled from the _____ through the cervix and out through the vagina.

chorionic

160. Thus, the consequent increase of uterine contractility and the onset of *labor* is related to (increasing/decreasing) levels of progesterone.

uterus

161. A few days after birth (called _____) *milk production* is initiated in the *mammary* glands.

decreasing

162. LTH regulates the initiation of *lactogenesis* or *milk* production by the mammary _____.

parturition

163. While the production of milk is called _____, milk *secretion* has the special term *galactopoiesis.*

glands

164. The continuation of galactopoiesis depends on adequate levels of STH, thyroxin, and adrenal cortical _____.

lactogenesis

165. In addition, emptying of the breast is essential to the continuation of milk secretion, or (galactopoiesis/lactogenesis).

    hormones

166. When the nipples are stimulated by suckling, nervous impulses are sent to the *posterior pituitary* by way of the central nervous system.

    Oxytocin is then released by the _____ pituitary.

    galactopoiesis

167. The posterior pituitary releases _____ thus causing muscle contractions in the mammary glands which expel milk.

    posterior

168. With the aid of muscle contractions, milk is expelled by the _____ glands. These contractions are caused by the hormone _____.

    oxytocin

169. Oxytocin is released in response to _____ impulses arising from the suckling stimulus.

    mammary
    oxytocin

170. In addition to their role in the menstrual cycle, the *estrogens* lead to the development of *secondary sex* characteristics in the female. Hair and fat distribution and development of the *mammary* glands

    are _____ _____ characteristics of the female.

    nervous

171. The male *testis* has two functions. In addition to the production of sperm, it performs the *endocrine* function of secreting androgens, or male sex

    _____.

    secondary sex

172. *Testosterone* is the most prominent male hormone,

    or _____.

    hormones

173. LH from the anterior pituitary gland stimulates testosterone production by the _____.

    androgen

174. Testicular secretion of _____   testis
begins at puberty and leads to the development of
male *secondary sex characteristics.*

175. Growth of facial hair, deepening of the voice, and   testosterone
prostate and penis development are examples of   (androgens)

     male _____ _____ characteristics.

     secondary sex

You have now completed the final section of Human Physiology. In this unit you
covered the functions and interrelations of one type of body glands known as endoc-
crine glands.

Before you take the final examination you may go back and review any section or
part of a section you wish.

REVIEW QUESTIONS

The following questions have been designed to guide your review of the programmed instruction in the human physiology course. You should not limit your
review to the areas covered in these questions, but they will serve to guide you in
determining the type of information you should assimilate.

REVIEW NUMBER ONE

The questions in this review section are based on the study of Sections I and II of
the programmed human physiology instruction.

Multiple-Choice Questions

In each of the following items, select the choice which most accurately completes
the statement or answers the question.

_____ 1. The extracellular fluids include (a) interstitial fluid; (b) plasma;
(c) special fluids; (d) all of the above.

_____ 2. Potassium ion (K^+) (a) is nearly 40 times more concentrated within
the cell than outside; (b) is about 12 times more concentrated within
the cell than outside; (c) is about 40 times more concentrated outside
the cell than inside; (d) is about 12 times more concentrated outside
the cell than inside.

_____ 3. Which of the statements in question 2 applies to the sodium ion (Na^+)?

_____ 4. Diffusion (a) is the flow of a substance from a region of higher concentration to a region of lower concentration; (b) is the flow of a substance from a region of lower concentration to a region of higher concentration; (c) is dealt with in Fick's law; (d) a and c.

_____ 5. The sodium leak refers to (a) the flow of Na^+ out of a cell; (b) the flow of Na^+ into a cell; (c) a and b; (d) none of the above.

_____ 6. Active transport (a) does not involve the expenditure of energy; (b) is made possible by the release of free energy when ADP is converted to ATP; (c) is made possible by the release of free energy when ATP is reconverted into ADP; (d) none of the above.

_____ 7. Osmosis (a) is a special case of diffusion; (b) is illustrated by the flow of water from a higher concentration to a lower concentration of water; (c) a and b; (d) none of the above.

_____ 8. Osmotic pressure varies directly with (a) the absolute temperature of the solution; (b) solute particle concentration; (c) a and b; (d) none of the above.

_____ 9. The permeability of a substance is related to its (a) lipid solubility; (b) molecular size; (c) electrical charge; (d) all of the above.

_____ 10. The word mole is a synonym for (a) ATP; (b) osmotic pressure; (c) gram molecular weight; (d) none of the above.

_____ 11. A solution with a greater osmotic pressure than another solution is (a) hyperosmotic; (b) isotonic; (c) isosmotic; (d) none of the above.

_____ 12. Which of the following statements is false? (a) acids, bases, and salts dissociate in solution; (b) 1 mole of NaCl per liter makes a 2 osmolar solution; (c) 1 mole of glucose per liter makes a 1 osmolar solution; (d) the formula to determine osmotic pressure is $\pi = CR/T$.

_____ 13. The individual concentrations of most substances inside and outside of the living cell (a) remain fairly constant; (b) are equal; (c) a and b; (d) none of the above.

_____ 14. Electromotive force is (a) an inverse function of current; (b) is a direct function of resistance; (c) a and b; (d) none of the above.

_____ 15. The section of a nerve where changes in membrane potential are occurring is called the (a) resting site; (b) action site; (c) potential site; (d) active site.

_____ 16. During the spike potential (a) the Na^+ and K^+ ions move down their concentration gradients; (b) the Na^+ and K^+ ions move up their concentration gradients; (c) Na^+ moves from inside to outside the cell; (d) none of the above.

_____ 17. Only a strong stimulus can excite a nerve in (a) the absolute refractory period; (b) the partially refractory state; (c) a and b; (d) none of the above.

_____ 18. The arrival of an impulse to a point on the nerve fiber involves a total change of potential of (a) 100 mv; (b) 50 mv; (c) 25 mv; (d) 10 mv.

_____ 19. The effectiveness of an electrical stimulus to a nerve fiber is a function of (a) the strength of the current; (b) the time over which the current is applied; (c) a and b; (d) none of the above.

_____ 20. ACh release is favored by the presence of (a) calcium ions; (b) magnesium ions; (c) a and b; (d) none of the above.

_____ 21. Curare (a) blocks nerve-muscle impulse transmission; (b) is sometimes used during surgery as a muscle relaxant; (c) a and b; (d) none of the above.

_____ 22. How much muscle tension would result from the stimulation of half of a muscle's fibers (relative to maximum tension)? (a) ¼ maximum tension; (b) ½ maximum tension; (c) maximum tension; (d) none of the above.

_____ 23. The contraction phase of a muscle fiber (a) lasts only a short time; (b) is followed by a relaxation phase; (c) a and b; (d) none of the above.

_____ 24. Myasthenia gravis (a) is characterized by extreme muscle fatigue; (b) could result from a decrease in muscle sensitivity to acetylcholine; (c) a and b; (d) none of the above.

_____ 25. Tetanus (a) is a neuromuscular disorder; (b) may be caused by the toxin of a bacillus; (c) a and b; (d) none of the above.

True–False Questions

Decide and indicate below whether each of the following statements is true or false. (Use a T or F.)

_____ 1. A living system may be considered a population of component cells.

_____ 2. The most general feature of cellular activity is the maintenance of a nonequilibrium relationship with the cellular environment.

_____ 3. One factor that would promote an equilibrium of intracellular substances with the cellular environment is the lack of permeability of the cell wall.

_____ 4. As the difference in concentration of a substance becomes greater the rate of diffusion becomes slower.

_____ 5. Increasing the thickness of the cell membrane will increase the diffusion flow.

_____ 6. The free energy for the sodium pump is derived from the metabolism of food by the cell.

_____ 7. The leak of a substance from a cell is an active process.

_____ 8. Osmotic forces play an important part in the movement and distribution of water across cell membranes.

_____ 9. Osmosis refers to diffusion restricted by a completely impermeable membrane.

_____ 10. Osmolarity refers to the number of moles of solute particles in a solution.

_____ 11. A temperature of $300°$ on the absolute scale is equivalent to a temperature of $20°C$.

_____ 12. Under comparable conditions the movement of water across the cell membrane is much more rapid than the movement of sodium or potassium ions.

_____ 13. One liter of a solution containing one mole of solute is a molar solution.

_____ 14. The function of a nerve fiber is to conduct impulses from one point to another.

_____ 15. If a stimulus is applied to the center of a nerve fiber, saltatory conduction will proceed in both directions to each end of the fiber.

_____ 16. Group C fibers are the fastest conductors.

_____ 17. The magnitude of a spike (action) potential depends on the magnitude of the stimulus causing the spike potential.

_____ 18. If a weak current requires a long time to initiate a response by a nerve, a strong current will require less time to initiate the same response.

_____ 19. Nerve fibers are classified according to velocity of impulse conduction.

_____ 20. The fibers that are called nonmyelinated are Group A fibers.

_____ 21. An axon normally carries impulses from the body of a nerve cell to a muscle cell.

_____ 22. A fibril is made up of bundles.

_____ 23. The energy for contraction comes from ATP.

_____ 24. Usually all motor units are in the contraction phase at the same time and in the relaxation phase at the same time.

_____ 25. The nerve cell axon leads from the spinal cord to the muscle which it serves.

Matching Questions

Match the term or terms on the left with the phrase at the right which is most closely associated with it.

Section I

_____ 1. physiology

(a) fluid lying in the spaces between cells

_____ 2. osmotic pressure

(b) the fluid, noncellular, part of the blood

_____ 3. interstitial fluid

(c) diffusion restricted by a semipermeable membrane

_____ 4. plasma

(d) the gas constant

_____ 5. special fluid

(e) having the same osmotic pressure as a second solution

_____ 6. concentration

(f) study of the function of living systems

_____ 7. osmosis

(g) having a lower osmotic pressure than another solution

_____ 8. R ($\pi = CRT$)

(h) amount per unit volume

_____ 9. isosmotic

(i) fluid found within the central nervous system

_____ 10. hypoösmotic

(j) force per unit area due to concentration difference

Section II

_____ 1. nodes of Ranvier

_____ 2. saltatory conduction

_____ 3. Group A fibers

_____ 4. Group B fibers

_____ 5. Group C fibers

_____ 6. all-or-none principle

_____ 7. rheobase

_____ 8. chronaxie

_____ 9. acetylcholine

_____ 10. myelin sheath

(a) the fastest conductors

(b) fibers do not transmit part of an impulse

(c) time necessary to cause excitation using a current strength of twice rheobase

(d) from one node of Ranvier to the next

(e) chemical which increases the membrane potential of the muscle cell membrane

(f) conduct impulses at an average rate of 4 m/sec

(g) insulator surrounding the motor nerve

(h) indentations on the myelin sheath

(i) minimum current strength needed to excite a given fiber

(j) slowest conductors of impulses

Additional Exercises

Do the following:

1. Explain the sodium pump theory.

2. Describe the processes of diffusion and osmosis.

3. What principles are expressed in Fick's law?

4. Describe the sequence of events following a stimulus to a nerve fiber.

5. Explain the all-or-none principle.

REVIEW NUMBER TWO

The questions in this review section are based on the study of Sections III and IV of the programmed human physiology instruction.

Multiple-Choice Questions

In each of the following items, select the choice which most accurately completes the statement or answers the question.

_____ 1. Nerves carrying information from the central nervous system are termed (a) motor nerves; (b) efferent nerves; (c) a and b; (d) none of the above.

_____ 2. Proprioceptors (a) are primarily pain receptors; (b) provide information about the position of joints; (c) a and b; (d) none of the above.

_____ 3. Destruction of the reticular formation in the brain leads to (a) a deep sleep; (b) greater sensibility to sensory stimuli; (c) a and b; (d) none of the above.

_____ 4. The time taken for a reflex to occur depends on (a) the speed at which the nerve impulse is carried by the neurons; (b) the time the impulse takes to jump from one neuron to another in the reflex pathway; (c) a and b; (d) none of the above.

_____ 5. The labyrinths (a) are unrelated anatomically to the cochlea; (b) are proprioceptors; (c) a and b; (d) none of the above.

_____ 6. Which of the following statements is false? (a) the semicircular canals are fluid-filled; (b) above the hair cells of the utricle and saccule are the ear stones or otoliths; (c) the utricle and saccule are not sensitive to changes in velocity; (d) when the head moves, the ear stones and gelatinous mass move the cilia of the epithelial cells.

_____ 7. Relative to an old lens the young lens (a) is more elastic; (b) tends to assume a more spherical shape; (c) a and b; (d) none of the above.

_____ 8. The rods (a) are special nerve cells located in the retina; (b) contain pigments which are sensitive to light; (c) a and b; (d) none of the above.

_____ 9. Hearing a sound depends on (a) its frequency; (b) its loudness; (c) a and b; (d) none of the above.

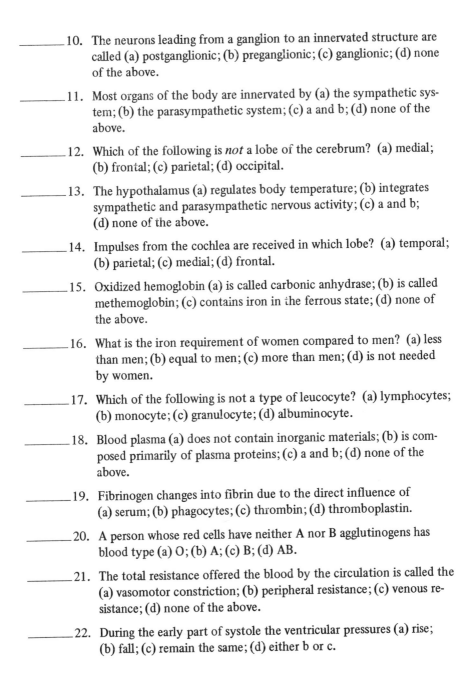

_____ 10. The neurons leading from a ganglion to an innervated structure are called (a) postganglionic; (b) preganglionic; (c) ganglionic; (d) none of the above.

_____ 11. Most organs of the body are innervated by (a) the sympathetic system; (b) the parasympathetic system; (c) a and b; (d) none of the above.

_____ 12. Which of the following is *not* a lobe of the cerebrum? (a) medial; (b) frontal; (c) parietal; (d) occipital.

_____ 13. The hypothalamus (a) regulates body temperature; (b) integrates sympathetic and parasympathetic nervous activity; (c) a and b; (d) none of the above.

_____ 14. Impulses from the cochlea are received in which lobe? (a) temporal; (b) parietal; (c) medial; (d) frontal.

_____ 15. Oxidized hemoglobin (a) is called carbonic anhydrase; (b) is called methemoglobin; (c) contains iron in the ferrous state; (d) none of the above.

_____ 16. What is the iron requirement of women compared to men? (a) less than men; (b) equal to men; (c) more than men; (d) is not needed by women.

_____ 17. Which of the following is not a type of leucocyte? (a) lymphocytes; (b) monocyte; (c) granulocyte; (d) albuminocyte.

_____ 18. Blood plasma (a) does not contain inorganic materials; (b) is composed primarily of plasma proteins; (c) a and b; (d) none of the above.

_____ 19. Fibrinogen changes into fibrin due to the direct influence of (a) serum; (b) phagocytes; (c) thrombin; (d) thromboplastin.

_____ 20. A person whose red cells have neither A nor B agglutinogens has blood type (a) O; (b) A; (c) B; (d) AB.

_____ 21. The total resistance offered the blood by the circulation is called the (a) vasomotor constriction; (b) peripheral resistance; (c) venous resistance; (d) none of the above.

_____ 22. During the early part of systole the ventricular pressures (a) rise; (b) fall; (c) remain the same; (d) either b or c.

_____ 23. Which of the following statements is false? (a) heart muscle normally contracts in a definite pattern; (b) it is possible for different parts of the heart muscle to depolarize out of phase; (c) blood flow is fairly constant throughout the systemic and pulmonary circulation; (d) if the veins are constricted, less blood is available to enter the ventricles.

_____ 24. Pressoreceptor impulses (a) inhibit the parasympathetic center in the medulla; (b) excite the parasympathetic center in the medulla; (c) excite the sympathetic center in the medulla; (d) a and c.

_____ 25. A decrease in blood pressure results from (a) a slowing of the heart; (b) vasodilation of the blood vessels; (c) a and b; (d) none of the above.

True-False Questions

Decide and indicate below whether each of the following statements is true or false. (Use a T or F.)

_____ 1. The motor nerve cells lie within the spinal cord.

_____ 2. There is a special nervous pathway leading to the central nervous system for each sensory receptor.

_____ 3. When a stimulus is continuously applied to a sensory receptor, the perceived sensation gradually increases.

_____ 4. In general, sensory information received on one side of the body goes to the sensory cortex on the same side of the brain.

_____ 5. Each motor neuron has a cell body located in the grey matter called an anterior horn cell.

_____ 6. The intrafusal muscles contract after stimulation by the gamma motor neuron.

_____ 7. When the body begins rotation, the fluid in the semicircular canal moves faster than the canal wall.

_____ 8. The ability of the eye to become more convex decreases with age.

_____ 9. The cochlea is divided by the stapes.

_____ 10. The utricle is continuous with the ends of each semicircular canal.

207

_____ 11. Sound vibration is transferred from the cochlea to the ossicles.

_____ 12. The energy of a sound is measured in cycles per second.

_____ 13. The pigment that enables red blood cells to carry oxygen is hemo-globin.

_____ 14. Broken down red cells are removed from the circulation by the reticulo-endothelial system.

_____ 15. The formation of prothrombin is increased by dicoumarol.

_____ 16. Transfusions of mismatched blood result in the clumping of the donated cells.

_____ 17. An increase in vasomotor activity decreases the radii of the arterioles.

_____ 18. The resistance to flow in a vessel is directly proportional to the cross-sectional area of that vessel.

_____ 19. Excitation of the heart muscle normally begins at the sino-atrial node.

_____ 20. The pressure in the left ventricle falls to the pressure level of the thorax during diastole.

_____ 21. Ventricular fibrillation speeds up blood flow.

_____ 22. The amount of blood that the large veins hold is regulated by the parasympathetic nervous system.

_____ 23. Impulses arriving over the vagus nerves cause the heart to speed up.

_____ 24. Pressoreceptor stimulation decreases blood pressure.

_____ 25. A person whose red cells have only agglutinogen A has type A blood.

Matching Questions

Match the term or terms on the left with the phrase at the right which is most closely associated with it.

Section III

_____ 1. localization

(a) neurons which release norepinephrine

_____ 2. muscle spindle

(b) brings about accommodation

_____ 3. accommodation

(c) neurons which release acetylcholine

_____ 4. ciliary muscles

(d) major site for interpreting sensory impulses

_____ 5. presbyopia

(e) intrafusal muscles together with the stretch receptor

_____ 6. adrenergic

(f) central area of the pons and medulla

_____ 7. cholinergic

(g) changing the power of the lens

_____ 8. reticular formation

(h) interprets visual stimuli

_____ 9. thalamus

(i) inability of the lens to increase its power

_____ 10. occipital lobe

(j) associating a sensation with a part of the body

Section IV

_____ 1. thrombus

(a) a narrowing of a valve orifice

_____ 2. stenosis

(b) sino-atrial node

_____ 3. fibrillation

(c) contraction phase

_____ 4. edema

(d) red cells are formed from these cells

_____ 5. hematopoetic factor

(e) relaxation phase

_____ 6. pacemaker

(f) intrinsic factor and vitamin B_{12}

_____ 7. systole

(g) clot occurring in the circulation

_____ 8. diastole

(h) results from low O_2 saturation of hemoglobin

_____ 9. cyanosis

(i) accumulation of fluid outside the circulation

_____ 10. reticulo-endothelial

(j) uncoordinated contractions of heart muscle

Additional Exercises

Do the following:

1. Describe a spinal reflex pathway.

2. Explain what is involved in a cross-extensor reflex.

3. List the major contents of blood plasma. Refer to Frame 59 of Section IV (the cardiovascular system) for the answer.

4. Describe the genesis of a red cell.

5. Discuss the meaning of one series of ECG waves labeled *PQRST*.

REVIEW NUMBER THREE

The questions in this review section are based on the study of Sections V, VI, and VII of the programmed human physiology instruction.

Multiple-Choice Questions

In each of the following items, select the choice which most accurately completes the statement or answers the question.

_____1. The fluid formed at the beginning of the nephron (a) is an ultra-filtrate of plasma; (b) is formed by the process of glomerular filtration; (c) a and b; (d) none of the above.

_____2. Which substance or substances appear(s) in the duct urine at a higher concentration than in the glomerular filtrate? (a) urea; (b) uric acid; (c) K^+; (d) all of the above.

_____3. Plasma clearance (a) varies inversely with the concentration of a substance in the urine; (b) varies directly with the concentration of a substance in the urine; (c) varies directly with the rate of urine flow; (d) b and c.

_____4. Which of the following statements is or are true? (a) the kidney regulates water and electrolyte concentrations of blood; (b) when glucose has a high concentration in the plasma, the tubular maximum may be exceeded; (c) a and b; (d) none of the above.

_____5. The renal response to increased PCO_2 of the blood is to (a) decrease secretion of H^+; (b) increase secretion of H^+; (c) decrease the re-absorption of HCO_3^-; (d) a and c.

_____ 6. Release of ADH is regulated (a) by impulses from osmoreceptor cells near the pituitary; (b) from blood volume receptors in the chest; (c) a and b; (d) none of the above.

_____ 7. Abnormal constituents of excreted urine include (a) protein; (b) glucose; (c) hemoglobin; (d) all of the above.

_____ 8. Which of the following is not one of the main classes of foods? (a) amino acids; (b) carbohydrates; (c) proteins; (d) fats.

_____ 9. The end products of protein digestion are (a) carbohydrates; (b) fats; (c) sugars; (d) amino acids.

_____ 10. Pertaining to the absorption of fat (a) all fat is absorbed as triglyceride; (b) some fat is absorbed as triglyceride; (c) no fat is absorbed as triglyceride; (d) all fat is absorbed as diglyceride.

_____ 11. Food in the duodenum initiates the release of (a) secretin; (b) pancreozymin; (c) a and b; (d) none of the above.

_____ 12. The main active ingredients of bile are (a) bile salts; (b) HCl; (c) droplets of fat; (d) none of the above.

_____ 13. The absorption of digested food occurs primarily in the (a) large intestine; (b) small intestine; (c) stomach; (d) none of the above.

_____ 14. Feces consists of (a) undigested food; (b) bacteria; (c) cellular fragments; (d) all of the above.

_____ 15. The variables used in describing changes in a gas are (a) pressure and volume; (b) pressure, volume, temperature, and number of moles; (c) pressure and temperature; (d) none of the above.

_____ 16. Of the total CO_2 transported in blood, most is in the form of (a) bicarbonate ions; (b) carbamino compounds; (c) carbonic acid; (d) none of the above.

_____ 17. The rate at which O_2 is supplied to the tissue capillaries depends upon (a) the amount of O_2 in the blood (combined with Hb); (b) the rate at which the heart pumps the blood to the tissues; (c) a and b; (d) none of the above.

_____ 18. Rhythmic breathing is controlled by nervous pathways originating in the (a) hypothalamus; (b) medulla; (c) pons; (d) b and c.

_____ 19. The external intercostals increase the volume of the thorax by moving the rib cage (a) upward and outward; (b) downward and inward; (c) upward and inward; (d) downward and outward.

_____ 20. Receptors sensitive to a large decrease in PO_2 are located in the (a) aorta; (b) carotid arteries; (c) pulmonary vein; (d) a and b.

Decide and indicate below whether each of the following statements is true or false. (Use a T or F.)

_____ 1. Blood flow through the glomerulus is regulated by constriction or dilation of its afferent and efferent arterioles.

_____ 2. Blood pressure is less than renal tubular pressure.

_____ 3. About 99% of filtered water is reabsorbed.

_____ 4. Na^+ is actively reabsorbed from the filtrate by both the proximal and the distal tubules of the nephron.

_____ 5. Decreased Na^+ reabsorption leads to an increased water reabsorption and diuresis.

_____ 6. A low pH indicates a low concentration of H^+ in the blood.

_____ 7. When the excretion of bicarbonate is high, the excretion of chloride is low.

_____ 8. Blood pH is regulated by the lungs and the kidneys.

_____ 9. Fats are composed of fatty acids and glycerol.

_____ 10. Stimulation of the sympathetic system increases intestinal peristalsis.

_____ 11. A salt that retains water in the intestine and thus acts as a laxative is magnesium sulfate.

_____ 12. Pancreatic juice does not contain enzymes.

_____ 13. An enzyme which breaks proteins into smaller molecules is pepsin.

_____ 14. Fat is transported to all parts of the body via the circulation of blood.

_____ 15. The alveoli of the lungs contain the same gases as are present in the atmosphere.

_____ 16. The pleural membranes lining the intrapleural space absorb gases but not fluids.

_____ 17. The muscles that increase the volume of the thorax by moving the rib cage are the internal intercostals.

_____ 18. The vital capacity varies with a person's age and the condition of his lungs.

Match the term or terms on the left with the phrase at the right which is most closely associated with it.

_____ 1. carbonic anhydrase   (a) usual end product of carbohydrate digestion

_____ 2. carbonic acid   (b) hormone which inhibits the activity of the stomach

_____ 3. carbamino compounds   (c) transport process that does not require cellular energy

_____ 4. tidal volume   (d) reabsorptive process that requires the expenditure of cellular energy

_____ 5. residual volume   (e) stimulates the secretion of pancreatic juice

_____ 6. vital capacity   (f) amount of air left in the lungs after a forced maximum expiration

_____ 7. lungs and kidneys   (g) dissociates into hydrogen and bicarbonate ions

_____ 8. ADH   (h) sugars and starches

_____ 9. passive   (i) regulate blood pH

_____ 10. active   (j) accelerates formation of carbonic acid

_____ 11. glucose   (k) causes the gall bladder to contract and discharge bile into the duodenum

_____ 12. carbohydrates   (l) volume of air normally inspired and expired

_____ 13. cholecystokinin   (m) formed by CO_2 combining loosely with hemoglobin and plasma proteins

_____ 14. secretin   (n) volume of air that can be expired after taking a full breath

_____ 15. enterogastrone   (o) controls water reabsorption in the distal tubule

Additional Exercises

Do the following:

1. Explain the Gas Law.

2. Describe what happens when CO_2 is dissolved in the blood.

3. Explain the functions of the hormones involved in the digestive process.

4. Describe glomerular filtration.

5. Describe bicarbonate reabsorption from the kidney tubule.

REVIEW NUMBER FOUR

The questions in this review section are based on the study of Section VIII of the programmed human physiology instruction.

Multiple-Choice Questions

In each of the following items, select the choice which most accurately completes the statement or answers the question.

_____ 1. Endocrine glands secrete (a) directly into the bloodstream; (b) externally; (c) hormones; (d) a and c.

_____ 2. The hypophysis (a) is another name for the pituitary gland; (b) consists of anterior and posterior portions; (c) a and b; (d) none of the above.

_____ 3. A deficiency of ADH (a) promotes an increased retention of water in the urine; (b) leads to diabetes insipidus; (c) a and b; (d) none of the above.

_____ 4. STH (a) is released by the anterior pituitary; (b) is the growth hormone; (c) a and b; (d) none of the above.

_____ 5. Which of the following statements is false? (a) an endocrine example of positive feedback is the relation between the thyroid gland and the pituitary gland; (b) TSH induces the thyroid gland to secrete thyroxin; (c) thyroxin is made from tyrosine and iodine in the thyroid gland; (d) thyroxin stimulates metabolism in all body tissues.

_____ 6. The body's basic energy requirement at rest is the (a) basal metabolic rate; (b) hypermetabolic rate; (c) isometabolic rate; (d) gross metabolic rate.

214

_____ 7. Goiter may be associated with (a) overactivity of the thyroid gland; (b) underactivity of the thyroid gland; (c) a and b; (d) none of the above.

_____ 8. The adrenal medulla secretes (a) epinephrine; (b) norepinephrine; (c) a and b; (d) none of the above.

_____ 9. The effect of epinephrine is to (a) decrease systolic blood pressure; (b) decrease heart rate; (c) decrease blood sugar; (d) none of the above.

_____ 10. Which of the following is not a class of steroid hormones produced by the adrenal cortex? (a) glucocorticoids; (b) beta steroids; (c) mineralocorticoids; (d) sex steroids.

_____ 11. Diabetes mellitus (a) is sometimes associated with hypersecretion of the glucocorticoids; (b) results from a deficiency of ADH from the anterior pituitary; (c) a and b; (d) none of the above.

_____ 12. The mineralocorticoids influence the kidneys to (a) excrete sodium; (b) reabsorb potassium; (c) a and b; (d) none of the above.

_____ 13. Addison's disease is characterized by (a) low blood pressure; (b) muscle weakness; (c) excessive loss of sodium chloride in the urine; (d) all of the above.

_____ 14. The ovaries produce (a) estrogens; (b) progestogens; (c) a and b; (d) none of the above.

_____ 15. Which of the following is not a phase of the menstrual cycle? (a) menstrual; (b) endometrial; (c) ovulatory; (d) progestational.

_____ 16. Oxytocin (a) is released by the posterior pituitary; (b) aids in the development of secondary sex characteristics in the female; (c) stimulates testosterone production; (d) none of the above.

_____ 17. Which of the following is not a male secondary sex characteristic? (a) galactopoiesis; (b) penis development; (c) prostate development; (d) growth of facial hair.

_____ 18. The adrenal medulla is activated by (a) low blood sugar; (b) fear; (c) low blood pressure; (d) all of the above.

_____ 19. The thyroid gland secretes (a) thyroxin; (b) epinephrine; (c) norepinephrine; (d) all of the above.

_____ 20. ACTH is produced by the (a) anterior pituitary; (b) posterior pituitary; (c) thyroid; (d) adrenal cortex.

True–False Questions

Decide and indicate below whether each of the following statements is true or false. (Use a T or F.)

_____ 1. Exocrine glands secrete externally.

_____ 2. Underactivity of the adrenal cortex is called Addison's disease.

_____ 3. Glucagon raises the blood sugar level.

_____ 4. In the liver amino acids are converted to glycogen.

_____ 5. Basal energy requirements are unrelated to a person's size.

_____ 6. Underactivity of the parathyroid gland leads to a decreased phosphate level in the blood.

_____ 7. In tetany there is an increased excitability of nerves.

_____ 8. Increased ACTH release leads to a decreased release of steroid hormones from the adrenal cortex.

_____ 9. STH is the growth hormone.

_____ 10. Underactivity of the thyroid gland is called hyperthyroidism.

_____ 11. Epinephrine and norepinephrine are known as catecholamines.

_____ 12. Aldosterone acts principally on potassium ion regulation.

_____ 13. The menstrual cycles cease during pregnancy.

_____ 14. The most prominent male hormone or androgen is testosterone.

_____ 15. ACTH stimulates the adrenal cortex.

_____ 16. The onset of labor is related to increasing levels of progesterone.

_____ 17. The placenta acts as an endocrine gland.

_____ 18. The endocrine glands are ductless.

_____ 19. One sysmptom of thyrotoxicosis is a BMR up to 50% below normal.

_____ 20. Hormones are secreted directly into the bloodstream.

Matching Questions

Match the term or terms on the left with the phrase at the right which is most closely associated with it.

_____ 1.	carpopedal spasms	(a) parturition
_____ 2.	chorion	(b) an increase in size of the thyroid gland
_____ 3.	childbirth	(c) secretes STH
_____ 4.	lactogenesis	(d) facilitates the intestinal absorption of calcium
_____ 5.	galactopoiesis	(e) secretes adrenal steroids
_____ 6.	ovulation	(f) may occur in tetany
_____ 7.	menstrual	(g) milk secretion
_____ 8.	goiter	(h) the release of an egg
_____ 9.	anterior pituitary	(i) secretes epinephrine
_____10.	posterior pituitary	(j) first phase of the menstrual cycle
_____11.	parathyroid	(k) milk production
_____12.	adrenal medulla	(l) secretes gonadotrophins
_____13.	adrenal cortex	(m) secretes PTH
_____14.	vitamin D	(n) secretes ADH
_____15.	placenta	(o) envelops the embryo

Additional Exercises

Do the following:

1. Can you name the phases of the menstrual cycle and describe the length and major events of each phase?

2. Describe the factors affecting blood calcium level.

3. Review the hormones produced by the anterior pituitary.

4. Do you remember the hormones produced by the adrenal cortex?

5. Describe the effects of epinephrine and norepinephrine.

ANSWERS TO REVIEW QUESTIONS

REVIEW NUMBER ONE

Multiple-Choice	True–False	Matching
		Section I
1. d	1. T	1. f
2. a	2. T	2. j
3. d	3. F	3. a
4. d	4. F	4. b
5. b	5. F	5. i
6. c	6. T	6. h
7. c	7. F	7. c
8. c	8. T	8. d
9. d	9. F	9. e
10. c	10. T	10. g
11. a	11. F	
12. d	12. T	
13. a	13. T	*Section II*
14. b	14. T	1. h
15. d	15. T	2. d
16. a	16. F	3. a
17. b	17. F	4. f
18. a	18. T	5. j
19. c	19. T	6. b
20. a	20. F	7. i
21. c	21. T	8. c
22. b	22. F	9. e
23. c	23. T	10. g
24. c	24. F	
25. c	25. T	

REVIEW NUMBER TWO

Multiple-Choice	*True–False*	*Matching*
		Section III
1. c	1. T	1. j
2. b	2. T	2. e
3. a	3. F	3. g
4. c	4. F	4. b
5. b	5. T	5. i
6. c	6. T	6. a
7. c	7. F	7. c
8. c	8. T	8. f
9. c	9. F	9. d
10. a	10. T	10. h
11. c	11. F	
12. a	12. F	*Section IV*
13. c	13. T	1. g
14. a	14. T	2. a
15. b	15. F	3. j
16. c	16. T	4. i
17. d	17. T	5. f
18. d	18. F	6. b
19. c	19. T	7. c
20. a	20. T	8. e
21. b	21. F	9. h
22. a	22. F	10. d
23. d	23. F	
24. b	24. T	
25. c	25. T	

REVIEW NUMBER THREE

Multiple-Choice	*True–False*	*Matching*
1. c	1. T	1. j
2. d	2. F	2. g
3. d	3. T	3. m
4. c	4. T	4. l
5. b	5. F	5. f
6. c	6. F	6. n
7. d	7. T	7. i
8. a	8. T	8. o
9. d	9. T	9. c

Multiple-Choice	True–False	Matching
10. b	10. F	10. d
11. c	11. T	11. a
12. a	12. F	12. h
13. b	13. T	13. k
14. d	14. T	14. e
15. b	15. T	15. b
16. a	16. F	
17. c	17. F	
18. d	18. T	
19. a		
20. d		

REVIEW NUMBER FOUR

Multiple-Choice	True–False	Matching
1. d	1. T	1. f
2. c	2. T	2. o
3. b	3. T	3. a
4. c	4. T	4. k
5. a	5. F	5. g
6. a	6. F	6. h
7. c	7. T	7. j
8. c	8. F	8. b
9. d	9. T	9. c
10. b	10. F	10. n
11. a	11. T	11. m
12. d	12. F	12. i
13. d	13. T	13. e
14. c	14. T	14. d
15. b	15. T	15. l
16. a	16. F	
17. a	17. T	
18. d	18. T	
19. a	19. F	
20. a	20. T	

INDEX

222

Iron, 99, 101
  ferritin, 102
Isometric muscle contraction, 56
Isosmotic solution, 23
Isotonic, muscle contraction, 56
  solution, 24

Ketone bodies, 186, 189
  ketosis, 186
Kidney(s), 150
  antidiuretic hormone (ADH), 162, 176
  blood pH, 160
  diuresis, 157
  nephrons, 150
  plasma clearance, 154
  reabsorption, 156, 187
  urine formation, 151

Labyrinths, 79
  fluid of, 81
  rotation principle, 81
Lens(es), 83
  accommodation, 83
  corrective, 85
  power of, 83
  system, 82
Leucocytes (white blood cells) 98, 103
  types, 103
Lipid solubility, 25, 27, 169
Liver, 102, 168
Living systems, 1-2
  organization, levels of, 1
Localization of sensation, 69
Logarithms, 144-145
Luteinizing hormone, 174, 176, 191,
  (LH, prolactin), 194
Luteotrophic hormone (LTH), 174, 176,
  191, 195
Lymphatic capillaries, 126

Malpighian corpuscle, 151
Medulla, 90, 92
  nerve impulse termination, 70
  pressoreceptors, 126
  respiratory center, 142
  vasoconstriction and vasodilation, 109,
    121
Membrane, cell, 5, 23
  composition of, 24
  impermeable, 7
  permeable, 7

Membrane (continued)
  pores, 25
  semipermeable, 15, 16, 23
Membrane potential, 36
  action potential, 39
  depolarization, 39, 49
  reduction of, 64
  resting, 39
Menopause, 193
Menstrual cycle, 191
Metabolism, food by cell, 9
  BMR, 180
  regulation, 186
  thyroxin, 180
Metabolites, 11
  efflux, 12
  influx, 12
Mineralocorticoids, 186-187
Mole, 19
Molecular size, 26
Motor cortex, 72, 95
Motor end plate, 48
  diagram, 48
Motor unit, 55, 57, 72
  nerve cell, body of, 58
Muscle, action potential, 49
  cardiac, 63
  cell, 31, 51
  contraction phase, 57
  external intercostal, 139
  function, loss of, 58
  intrafusal, 77
  involuntary (smooth), 185
    contraction of, 62
  relaxation phase, 57
  tone, 62
  voluntary (neuronal impulse), 72
    striated contraction, 52, 63
Muscle spindle, 77
  illustration, 78
Myelin sheath (nerve fiber), 41
  Ranvier, nodes of, 41
Myasthenia gravis, 58
Myofilaments, 51
Myosin filaments, 51, 55

Negative feedback, 178
Nephrons, 150
  illustration, 150
Nerve, afferent (sensory), 67, 88
  all-or-none principle, 42